Observations on the Nature of Gout, Ring-worm and Scarlet Fever

BY SAMUEL WESTCOTT TILKE,

MEDICAL HERBALIST.

2022 Transcription by J S Tilke

Published in 2023 by the transcriber, John Stuart Tilke

Tilke, Stuart
Observations on the Nature of Gout, Ring-worm and Scarlet Fever by Samuel Westcott Tilke, 2022 Transcription
ISBN: 9781447518716
    Imprint: Lulu.com

Autobiography/ Herbalism/ Botanical/ Victorian/ Sidmouth/ London/ Devon/ Medical/ Botanist/ Gout/ Scrofula/ Digestion/ Ringworm/ Scarlet Fever/ Scald-head/ Dropsy/ Medical Profession

OBSERVATIONS

ON

THE NATURE OF GOUT,

RING- WORM,

AND

SCARLET FEVER.

By S. W. TILKE,

1834.

OBSERVATIONS

ON THE

NATURE OF GOUT,

SHEWING

AN INFALLIBLE METHOD FOR ITS CURE.

ALSO

REMARKS

ON

DISEASES OF THE SCALP,

INCLUDING THE

RING-WORM.

TOGETHER WITH

SUGGESTIONS ON THE TREATMENT

OF THE

SCARLET FEVER.

By S. W. TILKE.

"And the Lord God planted a garden in Eden: and there He put the man whom He had formed. And out of the ground made the Lord God to grow every tree that is pleasant to the sight, and good." Gen. ii. 8. 9.
"And the fruit thereof shall be for meat, and the leaf thereof for medicine." - Ezek. xlvii. 12.

LONDON:

PRINTED BY J. POULTER, GT. CHESTERFIELD STREET.

1834.

"I pray thee understand a plain man,
In his plain meaning."
SHAKSPEARE.

NOTICE.

"I prattle out of fashion, and I dote
In mine own comforts."

                                    SHAKSPEARE.

The author of this work considers it his duty to impress on the minds of his readers, that he can only be seen at home between the hours of eight in the morning and three in the afternoon. From three to seven in the evening he visits, and from seven to twelve gives baths at home; therefore, every moment of time being fully engaged, this notice becomes highly necessary, especially as it frequently happens that patients come a great distance, and are disappointed at not having an interview. The author is strict to his time, as he considers punctuality and confidence necessary in all business, and it is each one's duty to comply: "pleasure in business make the hours seem short."

The author's fee for consultation at home is 3s. 6d.; out, under one mile, 7s.; under two miles, 10s. 6d.; and distance within the twopenny-post, £1. 1s.

CONTENTS.

Caution to Parents in their attempts to remove or check this disease; Cleanliness of the first importance; Truly dreadful consequence likely to ensue from some repelling applications; Author challenges the whole Faculty to cure the worst description of Scalled-head; This complaint admits of no uniform mode of treatment, members of the same family requiring different applications; Letters acknowledging the efficacy of the Author's treatment of this disease in all its varieties, in the most desperate cases; On Scarlet Fever, and the modern mode of treating this disease; The Author's ideas of this erroneous system of treatment, and suggestions to the Faculty.

"Were it possible for us to view through the skin and integuments, the mechanism of our bodies, after the manner of the watchmaker when be examines a watch, we should be struck with an awful astonishment! Were we to see the stomach and intestines busily employed in the concoction of our food by a certain undulatory motion; the heart working, day and night, like a forcing pump; the lungs blowing alternate blasts; the humours filtrating through innumerable strainers; together with an incomprehensible assemblage of tubes, valves, and currents, all actively and unceasingly employed in support of our existence, we could hardly be induced to stir from our places."

IGNOTUS.

"Strange! that a harp of thousand strings
Should keep in tune so long."

WATTS.

PREFACE

TO THE SECOND EDITION.

"We spend our days in unprofitable questions and disputations, intricate subtleties, about moonshine in the water, leaving, in the mean time, those chief treasures of nature untouched, wherein the best medicines for all manner of diseases are to be found: and do not only neglect them ourselves, but hinder, condemn, forbid, and scoff at others that are willing to inquire after them" –

Dr. Burton's Lectures.

In the Preface to the Second Edition of my work, I feel myself called upon to return thanks to the Almighty, for the numerous blessings he has showered on me since my first work appeared. When I consider the numerous difficult cases which have been placed under my care, many of which I have been induced to undertake only by the most urgent solicitation; and at the same time reflect that I have not only not failed in any single instance, but have been eminently successful in most; and that my efforts have been crowned with the approbation of all who have watched the progress of my establishment, together with the acknowledgments of my numerous patients and their friends, as to the efficacy of my mode of practice, I bow in grateful adoration to that Being who has seen fit that I should be instrumental in mitigating the load of suffering which mankind are doomed to bear from diseases incident to our nature.

Contrast this with what might by possibility have occurred had I failed in any case had any of the difficult cases placed in my hands, terminated fatally, what had I not to dread, previously to my being so generally known to the public? And yet how possible was this failure, when in many instances patients have come to me only at the eleventh hour. The plain reason which may be assigned for this uniform success is, that my practice may *mitigate*, but cannot *aggravate*. Disease may be driven out -the blood may be purified, lameness removed, morbific humours expelled, the whole system restored to healthy action; but by no possibility can these complaints be, aggravated, or driven in, for any the least *tyro* will soon perceive, on reading the following pages, or visiting my establishment, that all my efforts are directed to the *removal* of complaints, not the mere mitigation of them. And it can as easily be perceived, that the medicines used must be of the most harmless (although powerful) nature: so simple are they, that the patient is not restricted in diet, beyond the observance of moderation; very little internal medicine, and this generally decoctions of the most simple herbs, such as I have recommended in this work, in addition to many others too numerous to name.

If those abominable ingredients, mercury, colchium, pruissic acid, with a long list of other *poisons*, the names of which are to be found in every pharmacopeia, were the means I used for these cures, the end might probably soon be apparent. But let no dissimulation be used. There are herbs and roots to be gathered in different parts of England, possessing all the power, without the deleterious effects of the above miserable minerals. Who can calculate the numbers which have been hurried to an untimely grave by this sad preference given to minerals!

Let not the use of VEGETABLE MEDICINE be called an innovation - this was the practice of olden times, when disease was not near so prevalent, and when, so well known were the properties of herbs and roots, that every village had its *Dame*, equal to the ordinary cases of indisposition which occurred, and *Doctors* were called in much less frequently than in our days, when a child cannot cut its teeth, or an adult have an attack of *bile*, but the medical practitioner must be called in. The change has been gradual, and at last so general has it become, that he who asserts there are growing in England herbs sufficient for most pharmaceutical purposes, is said to be dealing in mysteries. No doubt, the difficulty would be great to restore at once the use of herbs, in place of minerals, especially as the public generally enquire little for themselves in these matters, leaving it to the faculty. Let any one expect the change from the faculty, and they will be deceived: First, their trade thrives much better as it is. And though there are a very numerous portion of liberal-minded men in the profession who would gladly adopt any change, which might prove beneficial to mankind, yet they have not the power - they are completely under a set of *rules*, to differ from which would most certainly be their ruin. This we well know, from what has happened; not a few celebrated men could be named who have been *cut*, for daring to think and act upon what their good sense might shew them to be superior. This is a subject deeply to be regretted, especially at a time when several diseases stalk through the land, without even the pretension of a cure - witness consumption - gout - cholera, &c. &c.. Surely this is a time to ask for *new lights*, not to check by Parliamentary regulations the persevering efforts of individuals to undermine disease.

What can be more absurd, at a period when every species of knowledge and science is by the medium of the public press daily subjected to the scrutiny of millions of British eyes, than the practice of the physicians of England, pertinaciously to adopt an unintelligible foreign *dead tongue*, instead of the *living language* of their own country! *First*, because scarcely any two of them use the same Latin words, in a prescription for the same thing. – *Secondly*, because if they have had a classical education, to qualify them to write Latin correctly, it is obvious that their prescriptions must be entrusted to young men generally to dispense, whose age renders it impossible that they should clearly understand them.

Again, with respect to the far greater mass of medical practitioners, the *apothecaries*, how grossly vicious is the present system! They are not paid by the benefit conferred on their patients, neither for their attendance bestowed on them; but by the number of bottles and boxes of pills which their skill can contrive to send every day. Even in that most interesting science of anatomy and surgery it is to be hoped, whilst it is making such rapid advancement throughout Europe, that our lectures will daily become more intelligible to the public mind.

It would be too much for me to calculate on invariable success or pretend to infallibility - should any sufferer persist, as a last resource, in placing himself in my hands, and I undertake his case, hoping there still may remain a remote chance of snatching him from death - and yet the King of Terrors should ultimately prevail, when

"It is too late; the life of all his blood
Is touched corruptibly: and his pure brain
(Which some suppose the soul's frail dwelling-house)
Doth, by the idle comments that it makes,
Foretell the ending of mortality."
SHAKSPEARE.

am I to expect the reproaches of the Profession and the Public? Let it be understood that every practical man must have many cases terminate fatally under his hands every year. Let them visit my house, question my patients, acquaint themselves with my system, and judge how far I experimentalize, so that should any case end fatally, they may be able to depose how far *my* treatment was good or otherwise for be it observed, I solicit the visits of those medical gentlemen who may at any time have attended the patients coming to my establishment - they may there daily watch the progress of the cure - and judge how far the treatment is judicious or otherwise. This I am happy to say is very frequently done, and I feel desirous that all who can spare the time, will examine for themselves. After this, I trust I shall have the credit given me of acting openly and candid.

Many remarks on *the Profession* in this work may be thought too harsh - but I wish them to be understood as applying to those who object to any improvement on the system - such as pertinaciously adhere to their own beaten track, and treat such efforts as mine with contumely. Such persons I have encountered:

> "Where I have seen them shiver and look pale,
> Make periods in the midst of sentences,
> Throttle their practis'd accent in their fears,
> And, in conclusion, dumbly have broke off,
> Not paying me a welcome. Trust, me, sweet,
> Out of this silence yet I pick'd a welcome,
> And in the modesty of fearful duty
> I read as much as from the rattling tongue
> Of saucy and audacious eloquence."
>
> SHAKSPEARE.

I feel bound to esteem the respectable practitioner - of many of whom, from experience, I have reason to speak in the highest terms, and am proud to rank amongst my best friends. Indeed, so far has liberality of feeling been extended towards me, that in an interview of nearly an hour with His Majesty's Medical Board, by appointment, their unqualified approval of my answers to their questions on professional subjects, were expressed in such kind language as will never be forgotten by me; nothing could have more strengthened me in my present pursuits, than the repeated approbation of so enlightened a body as constituted this Board. Many others have kindly taken a daily interest in my welfare. And, surely, I must be ungrateful in the extreme, did I not in the most public manner express my sense of their kindness. I cannot too distinctly declare, there fore, that my remarks are meant only to apply to the illiberal and unenlightened.

I fear there may be found much in the following pages uninteresting to a general reader, especially those parts relating to myself. But it must be borne in mind, that in some companies when my name is introduced in conversation, the first question is, "who is he?" - This must be my apology for placing my self so prominently before the public.

I trust this work will not be subjected to severe criticism; it has been hastily thrown together, in the midst of important avocations, and would hardly have met the public eye, but at the request of friends, to whose wishes I was induced to comply.

In days when Quackery may perhaps exist to an injurious extent, I am anxious to shew, that I am not a needy adventurer, bent upon my own aggrandizement, but filling an ostensible situation in society, rather thrust into it, than seeking it for myself. If success had not attended my progress, I should calmly have returned to my original pursuit, and endeavoured to retain the character for integrity which I always possessed; but since I have been blessed with success in such a remarkable degree, I should be not less a traitor to the Public than to myself, were I to relinquish my present pursuits.

Deeply grateful to those who have extended to me their friendship, and to those, much my superiors, who who have kindly admitted me on their list of friends,

I subscribe myself,

Their most obedient humble servant,

S. W. TILKE.

No. 8, Thayer Street.
Jan. 1st, 1834

PREFACE

TO THE FIRST EDITION.

In offering my services to the Public, through the medium of the few pages contained in this pamphlet, it will be easily discovered that I have not the least pretension to the rank of medical science, but that I appear before the world as a plain, humble, and I trust, too, honest man; induced by no motive to become conspicuous, but that of doing good to my fellow creatures.

By a perusal of the following pages, it will be seen how, and in what manner, the first seeds of my medical knowledge were sown; how these were afterwards nursed, reared, and brought to maturity; and the testimonials of the highly respectable individuals that follow, will shew also the happy results arising from my exertions.

I have stated above, that I pretend not to the high rank of medical science, and when I at the same time am enabled to state, that Providence has so blessed my early efforts in life, as to make pecuniary affairs of really secondary importance, I trust it will be inferred that I *deserve no rank* with those low, sordid, ignorant pretenders, whose only object is to enrich themselves at the sacrifice of the health and lives of their victims; and I take this opportunity of declaring, that it never was any part or plan of my intentions to intrude myself on public notice in connexion with the healing art, but that having, at various periods of my life, for charity's sake alone, prescribed my remedies for the poor and destitute, without fee or reward, and every case terminating in perfect recovery, continually led to new applications, till nearly the whole of my time was occupied, to the neglect of my more immediate pursuit, imperceptibly leading me to that in which I now publicly offer my services. The late noble and generous-minded Lord Robert Seymour was in the frequent habit of administering pecuniary support to those poor afflicted persons who have at various times been under my medical care, and thus gave me the most gratifying support.

Having been thus led step by step to endeavour to alleviate the sufferings of my fellow-creatures, I have at length been induced, by the repeated intreaties of my friends, to take a suitable residence, where I might with more convenience to myself, and comfort to my patients, receive those who honour me with their confidence; and I have only to add, that, urged by a sense of duty, I shall now devote the whole of my time to that study, by the constant success of which I have reason to hope for encouragement in my future progress.

No. 8, Thayer Street, Manchester Square.
July 1831

ON THE

NATURE AND TREATMENT

OF

GOUT.

"A plague of this gout, or a gout of this plague; for the one or the other plays the rogue with my great toe."

SHAKSPEARE.

In offering my services to the Public, with the bold assertion that I possess the certain means of curing that hitherto styled *incurable* malady, the Gout, it will be said by many, especially by interested persons, that it is an attempt at imposition, for the purpose of filling my own pockets at the expense of the credulous; and that I am an empiric, equal with, and as much to be avoided, as the many who so dishonourably subsist by vile and disgraceful pretensions. I have always considered

What is easily earned, is easily lost,
For ill got wealth is at the owner's cost.

But as I have full confidence in the motto, "that truth conquers all things," and possessing at the same time (as a result from my practice) the privilege to refer to hundreds of living witnesses, that what I assert is *true*, I have no reason to care for either the malice or the jealousy of any, but shall fearlessly and perseveringly pursue my plan of treatment; being well assured that, under the guidance of Providence, I shall be instrumental in rescuing many of my fellow-creatures from a repetition of the most agonizing affliction to which human nature is liable. Various and combating, indeed, are the opinions of medical men, both as to the precise nature and the treatment of Gout; and perhaps too, no disease ever gave rise to more speculative theory on the one hand, and more industry on the other, to endeavour to find a remedy, even if it were only a temporary relaxation from suffering, but all in vain; and Gout is allowed, for the want of means to prevent it, to run its course, or as it is usually termed, - to be laid up with a *fit* of the Gout.

The Profession consider it as a disease above their range, and of a nature not to be meddled with without the greatest risk of doing more harm than good: they consider the Gout, as a Physician sent by Nature to torture the poor patient, but at the same time, to destroy all the other diseases of his mortal body. Reader, tell me what think you, if this is the only perfection to which they have brought medical knowledge during so many years! Do the savages of Africa or America furnish us with greater absurdities than these? Read what a learned Doctor has lately written on the subject of Gout. Dr. Sutton, after speaking upon the disease with all his scientific knowledge, owns that *"the only advance made in the knowledge of the treatment of Gout has been by Quacks; that is to say, Quacks and Empirics have led the way to Physicians, Doctors, Physiologists, and Pathologists."* If this be true, what have the Professors of the boasted sciences of Anatomy, Surgery, and Pathology been about? Was it not their place to have found out, and not required the assistance of *Quacks*? If this be the doctrine in the School of Medicine, they may in truth be called schools. Why remain school-boys all their lives! Now, Dr. Wilson is the proprietor of a Quack Medicine; I suppose that, being a member of the Royal Medical Society of Edinburgh, and Graduate of the same, he is not well pleased at the Profession calling him a plain *Quack*. Suppose we call him a *Medico Quack*, or *Quack Medicus*. However, though he may have drawn on himself the wrath of his medical brethren, he does not seem to feel much concern, for he tells them in good set terms that they are all *Quacks*, as they make use of ingredients they know not the properties of, or from whence they come. Perhaps, their answer would be, *"We must take, and use the Profession as we found it; if people will be sold, they must be bought there is now no living without it."*

"Oh place! oh form! how often doth thou with thy ease, thy habit, wrench awe from fools; and tie the wiser souls to thy false seeming!"

What could *Shakspeare* mean by this? Again - Dr. Badlam, Professor of Medicine in Glasgow, in a recent lecture, says, *"One of these days I mean to introduce the dear public to the examining schools; the dear public now go every where ; they go to Almack's and to the Drawing- room: why not show them how doctors are made, a process in which they are certainly a good deal interested; indeed it were well that the Public knew better than it does, of what stuff a considerable number of our medical alumnia is actually composed."* Again he says, *"A slight reference to ancient medicine is also positively useful; because, to mark progress we must have the point of departure; because it is well to know how much was accomplished with very limited means; because we can only in this manner trace the introduction of new medical agents; and because it is not uninstructive to mark how old things again become new"* I wish a few more would confess this much, and change their practice.

Dr. Buchan says, *"Fashion reigns in physic with as arbitrary a sway as in dress; and there is no disease which shews the imperfection of medicine in a stronger light than the Gout. Many things will shorten a fit, - and some will drive it off altogether, but nothing has yet been found which will do this with safety, and a patient will hazard life itself for a temporary relief."* And *"It would be as imprudent to stop the Small-Pox from rising, and to drive them into the blood, as to attempt to repel the gouty matter."* With this I agree. Again he says, *"The instruments of medicine will always be multiplied in proportion to men's ignorance of the nature and causes of diseases. When these are sufficiently understood, the method of cure will be simple and easy; for the study of nature is simply spirit and intelligence."*

It cannot be expected that I should divulge the system of cure of which I am in possession, for the benefit of professional gentlemen, who cannot but acknowledge themselves ignorant on this branch of medical science; and who are not sufficiently spirited or generous to make or offer a competent remuneration to obtain it: for on those terms I offered it, long before those friends I had cured made it publicly known, as I had then other occupations. And to shew that I had no wish to be seen in the practical part of my own inventions, will be proved by the following fact. One day, while in conversation with a medical gentleman respecting my pursuits, I told him if I did not soon have an offer from a medical man, to introduce my system into practice, I should consider myself in duty bound, by every principle of nature, morality, and religion, either to do so myself, or cause it to be done by some non-professional ma ; but that, if he would undertake it, and allow me £50 a-year for as many years as he cleared £500, I would immediately put him in possession of every information to enable him to do so. I will now give his answer almost to the very letter: *"I am convinced, Mr. Tilke, it would be for the interest of both, as well as that of the public, could I comply with your proposition; but consider, the whole of the profession, when it came to their knowledge, would stamp me a quack, and shun me; by such means what little practice I now have I should soon lose."* I am very sorry my friend still remains with a *little practice*, and what is worse, a very large family; he has since repeatedly expressed his deep regret at having clung to the shadow and lost the substance, and has repented it ever since.

To those who accuse me of pirating from the Profession, I would ask, have they not themselves set me the example? Do not the Druggists pirate from the Apothecary, the Apothecary from the Physician, the Physician from the Surgeon, and the Surgeon from the whole of them? Are they not at this moment applying to the Legislature to prevent their Scottish brethren from participating in the same privileges as themselves? - by doing which, are they not turning their lancets and scalpels against each other, and converting what ought to be a peaceful lecture-room, into a field of battle, and lowering the respectability of science, for the gratification of petty jealousy and private malice? It were better the profession were at once thrown open to a fair competition of skill and talent. However, I have no wish to destroy or disturb the different orders of the profession; I only wish to bring them back to the spirit for which their institution was first intended. I will just give this friendly hint: if they do not mind, while they are quarrelling about the bone, other men of more liberal practice, will run away with the meat; as Shakspeare says -

> For every order includes itself in power,
> Power into will - will into appetite;
> And appetite - an universal wolf,
> So doubly seconded with will and power,
> Must make, perforce, an universal prey,
> And last, eat up *himself.*

My medical as well as non-medical friends have heard me express the same opinion for the last fifteen years; and could I have found any man in the profession who would have acted on my suggestions, and practised with my very simple vegetable medicine, I should now have been in that humble, though respectable, situation of life in which I was originally placed, and in which fortune smiled on me. But I should have been wanting in duty to my fellow-creatures, after having failed in my endeavours with the profession to adopt my system of cure, had I not put my inventions in practice; though it was at that time to leave a certainty for an uncertainty. What has it done for me? Why, given me an introduction to an elevated class of society, and to the personal confidence and friendship of a class of men, whom, from my retired habits, I should never otherwise have been introduced to. Many of those who laughed at my *"ideas,"* now, I have no doubt, seeing my success, begin to think, that a wise man may make use of that which none but a fool could have invented. To the idle and envious part of the profession, who would ridicule and hinder those that labour for the public, though they themselves have not the ability equal to do the same, may go on and think as their malignant nature inclines them. Such I would advise to pursue the path which Dame Nature hath designed them for; and let him whose only fault is that he entered the house of the profession, not with a diploma key, but by climbing up and getting in at the window - I say, let such have a fair trial of public opinion, and rise or fall according to the merits of his own invention; for all men have a just right to the instruction, benefit, and exercise of their own minds. All will find there is a book of nature in which the wisdom and power of the Almighty may be studied with scarcely any inferior edification. But it often happens that a scholar, with his systems and scientific methods, which *frequently overstep themselves*, finds himself stopt short when he attempts to study Nature; while the rustic, or untaught youth, furnished with Nature's key, is enabled to unlock every door of knowledge. All men would do well to consider that they will have to give in their account of their use or abuse of those talents which Nature hath given them, for where much is given, much will be expected.

The knowledge of remedies, without a previous knowledge of the precise nature and situation of disease, is an acquisition likely to lead persons into dangerous, and perhaps fatal consequences; but at the same time it is lamentable to say, that it forms the groundwork of the practice of many, who support themselves by trifling with the lives of their fellow creatures in this way.

The practice which I pursue for the cure of the Gout is of the most simple nature; but simple as it may be, it could never have been attained, had I not in early life been led by strong inclination to the study of botanical medicine. Fortunately for myself and my patients one discovery led to another.

The question perhaps may arise: What knowledge can I have of disease, or the internal part of man, not possessing a *diploma*, or having studied anatomy? To such I would reply, that for the last twenty years, I have had constant access to one of the finest anatomical museums this or any other country can boast of, where I received *advantages* equal with those who have passed through their regular degrees; and am proud to say, that I can reckon among my instructors and supporters some of the Profession, who have not only, from their knowledge of my practice, recommended me patients afflicted with Gout and Ringworm, but have even placed members of their own families under my care; and others have candidly admitted themselves converts to my opinion, as to the cause and cure of the Gout and Rheumatism. I will illustrate this by the following fact, the truth of which is easily ascertained, although it is not my object or practice to publish the names of my patients without their free consent; but of this and every other statement I make, I will afford to the curious an abundant means of arriving at the truth, on personal application.

About two years since, a first-rate physician sent for me. When I entered his room, he thus addressed me, taking me by the hand: *"Mr. Tilke, I have heard, through a medical friend, of the wonderful cure you have made on Captain (Blank), and other eminent persons, and am induced to send for you, having heard, after strict inquiry, of your natural bent for study, your ideas and modes of cure of the complaint with which I am now suffering. Whether your father made you a baker, tinker, or tailor, Nature intended your for the study of her works; and to shew you I mean what I say, it is my intention to place myself under your care; if you will attend me personally, and treat me as you would one who knew nothing of medicine, you shall say Dr. (Blank) is one of your best patients in attending to your directions."*

After my attendance on this gentleman, (who had been confined eleven months to his room with Gout,) for eight days, he sent a message to the wife of the gentleman who introduced me to him, that *"in one week more he should be able to walk her round Hyde Park."* From the success of this cure, I am proud to say, I have had some of the first Lords of the land place themselves under my care. Having thus much of private practice, and other pursuits that require my attention, I trust is sufficient answer to the inquiries of those who wonder I do not make my remedies more generally known by advertisements.

It may be thought by many strange that I should have discovered a remedy for two incurable diseases; some think it yet more strange that persons who profess to have studied to alleviate the sufferings of their fellow creatures, should assert there is any disease for which Nature has not provided a remedy. Acting upon this principle, I have spent all my leisure hours in retirement from the fatigues of business. Many of my intimate friends can bear me out, that after I had performed a cure for Ring-worm, about ten years since, I then said, I should never rest satisfied until I had succeeded in the discovery of a cure for the Gout, which has taken me many years to bring to its present perfection. I feel convinced that I have been directed by the hand of Providence, otherwise, from the many tedious processes I have had to travel through, I must have given it up in despair, and failed my desired object. But the Almighty has been pleased to bless me with an active, enterprizing mind; therefore I claim no credit to myself, believing, in the words of the immortal bard, *"that it has pleased Fate to bless me with this, and this with me;"* for:-

> "By a disease, when Nature's hard beset,
> She fights her foe, with labour, toil, and sweat,
> Her handmaid Herbs then to the battle flies,
> To her mistress' arms, and succours with supplies.
> Her aid by Heaven is blest, she bears the shield;
> But 'tis Dame Nature that disputes the field."

Dr. Potter says, *"There is a morbid matter in the Gout, but of what kind we are utterly ignorant; and that all gouty persons breed stone."* Dr. Allen confesses that the art of healing makes but slow advances towards perfection. *"There appears,"* he says, *"now and then, a person of extraordinary faculties and singular endowments, who in this most beneficial branch does signalize himself; but those men whom Nature hath peculiarly qualified, make but a small number."* Again, he says, *"The primary causes of disease are of so hidden a nature as to exceed any researches or penetration of mine; and, were we ingenuous in our confessions, they for the most part escape our inquiry. We sail, as it were, on the bosom of the mighty deep, unacquainted with the longitude."*

If we consider Nature we shall often find very contrary effects flow from the same cause: for instance, *Gout*, which seems chiefly to be the extravasation of *nervous fluid*; which with the *blood*, being over-heated, soon becomes impure, and forms a fluid or matter in the urinary organs, as well as in the liver, which soon makes them become sluggish in their operations. The liver also being larger in *man* than in any other living creature, considering the size of his body, subjects him to innumerable maladies. By the best experiments ever made, the blood is proved to consist of phlegm, spirits, oil, salt, and earth; but is professionally divided into serum and crassamentum, the former being the thin, fluid-like portion, and the latter the solid congealed-like cake; and the word *humours* is so indeterminate amongst many as hardly to have any meaning in it; but in general it contains this supposition, viz. that there is a faulty quality in that to which this name is given. Gouty humours, for instance, is another term for a diseased fluid; but the blood is the general humour or fluid from whence all the other humours or fluids in the body are separated; for without this knowledge of the particular humour or fluid, a man must be ignorant of the proper method of altering either the quantity or quality of the impurities of the blood, which I am sorry to say is too often brought on by those persons, and handed down to posterity, by the continual use of spirituous liquors, by always sipping, as it were, a liquid fire, which destroys digestion. The solids become impaired, the juices corrupted; and after the dreadful sufferings which such conduct brings on them, they are no sooner well, but they again prostitute their health, and run into the very arms of death. I do not mean to infer that all sufferers with Gout court this kind of destruction, because I know to the contrary, and have, in another part of this work, shewn that with some it is hereditary. On this point doctors differ; but Nature has so ordained it, that the opinions of men should not be the same. I must confess I have reaped the greatest advantage from reading and studying the works of those from whom I entirely differed: for I always read with my pencil in my hand, and I make marks and remarks as I go on. And although I may deliver my opinions in an imperfect manner, yet I trust that others may take advantage of my labours. May God, the eternal and inexhaustible source of all blessings, to whose goodness the success of all medicinal skill and application is entirely owing, favour my endeavours, that what ideas I have collected from others or learned from my own study and experience, may tend to the welfare of suffering mankind, whom I only ask to use my medicine until they find a better.

There is a prevailing opinion that a fit of the Gout is salutary to the system, and relieves it from other disorders. This I consider to be a fallacy: repeated attacks frequently produce debility both of body and mind, and the prevailing modes of treatment too often increase the violence of the disease. Dr. Cullen says there is no morbid matter present in per sons who have the Gout, and that the disease generally attacks those persons who have enjoyed the best health. My opinion is, that *Gout*, as it is termed, is not the work of a day; the causes are gradually accumulating, however suddenly the attack may be. The dam of these humours, *which has been shut up*, gives way, and bursts forth by an effort of nature to free herself from an offending cause. Then it becomes the duty of the attendant to observe with the greatest care and attention which way nature points, and assist her in her operations to expel or throw off whatever is injurious to health. I have noticed this disease attack the young and aged very differently, and I think for this good reason: in youth or prime of life the fibres are lax and soft, the nerves possess greater sensibility, and the fluids of more rapid motion: whereas in old age the fibres are rigid, the nerves become almost insensible, and many of the vessels inactive and perfectly useless, therefore of course they require more time and persevering of treatment. Many of my patients are able to bear me out when I state that a morbific matter has exuded through the skin, to a surprising extent; and this of great consistency, and which, before extraction, I think had been corroding in the urinary channels, preventing the free circulation. How can it be for a moment supposed, that the blood can be in a pure state, while the patient labours under Gout or Rheumatism!

Others contend that heat encourages the complaint. My practice entirely disproves this notion; my medicines cause a free circulation of blood by being internally and externally applied, and brings on a general in crease of action. Gout, from being treated improperly, is often diverted from its regular course, to the imminent danger of the patient. Those who do not inherit, or have not had the Gout, if they breed bad blood, have reason to expect it. And those who have an hereditary claim to this complaint, may by precautions as regards diet, guard themselves from its attacks.

I have before shown that other diseases arise from the same cause as the Gout; as Chronic Rheumatism, which sometimes affects the lumbar region so severely, that the patient cannot stand upright. This affliction is known by the name of Lumbago. Sometimes it fixes in the hip joint, and is then called *Sciatica*. All those affections or symptoms are to be treated nearly in the same manner as the Gout. Dr. Darwin mentioned it as a common opinion, that Gout is as frequently the consequence of gluttony as drunkenness.

Complaints are brought on by the improper use of drugs, given too frequently for the purpose of increasing fees, or multiplying the items of an apothecary's bill; the poor patient swallows every thing given him, without daring to ask the necessity or quantity of the dose. Many of the faculty are, no doubt, worthy of all the confidence that can be reposed in them, and have made the alleviation of human infirmity the principal study of their lives; unlike those who condemn that which they do not understand. The Faculty should reflect on the many discoveries yet to be made in the botanical world, where nothing grows in vain; but these virtues are, in general, unknown, or, rather say, neglected and abused, when they might be usefully employed as remedies to counteract the ills of human life. For instance, in the Royal Cabinet of Paris there are arrows whose points are impregnated with the juice of so venomous a plant, that with the slightest puncture they will destroy the stoutest animal that exists, as the blood of the victim instantly congeals; but if a small quantity of the juice of another plant be immediately taken, the circulation is as quickly restored. Both the poison and the remedy were discovered by the most uncivilized beings. I could enumerate hundreds of other similar cases, but that would be departing from my present object, viz. to shew the great neglect of medicinal herbs in the modern pharmacopoeia. There are not in the present day above two thousand, the properties of which are generally known; but if we read of olden times, when drugs were hardly known, the celebrated LINNÆUS gives the properties of from seven to eight thousand; the famous Sherard was acquainted with sixteen thousand; and another botanist speaks of from twenty to twenty-five thousand. Nature is of infinite extent, who invites to the study of her works men of every age, country, and condition of life. Her treasures are not confided to genius alone; but some and many of her fruits are reserved for the less literary and less informed. As a proof, how often does it happen that old women in the country, without education, by the help of a simple herb, gathered in its bloom, when it possesses its greatest strength and virtues, perform very extraordinary cures, in cases where the regular practitioner is absolutely at a loss how to treat them. I would not be understood to cast any reflections on the character of surgery; for a surgeon is like a guardian angel, who steps forward to alleviate the accidents of the unfortunate.

Dr. Squirrel says, *"Nothing can be more illiberal than the epithet of quack, when applied to those who retain the secret of their own discoveries."* On this head Sir Joseph Banks observes - *"I have no doubt that a medicine will prove more beneficial to the public when confined to the practice of an individual. It escapes the risk of being decried by theoretical persons, if the composition had been communicated to the faculty."* Dr. Squirrel again says, *"Whatever discoveries any man may make, are they not as much his property as the estate be purchases? Has society any right to enjoy the benefit of any person's labour or invention, without bis being rewarded in turn; and is there any other mode of rewarding the discoverer, but by keeping it a secret? Can remuneration be more equitable than when received from the individuals who receive the benefit? Is this not the principle on which the intercourse of society should be conducted through life, that is to say, mutual interest?"* The late Dr. Burnet says: - *"In whatever sphere of life an individual may be destined to move, if honest integrity attends him, and a full consciousness that he has, with the most scrupulous exactitude, fulfilled and substantiated the character which he professes to maintain, then he may, without presumption, lay claim to that reward to which his skill and exertions so justly entitle him."* In the environs of London we possess botanic gardens, kept up at a great expense, but unfortunately more for ornament than use. Nature has distributed her favours in every lane, field, and pathway, and affords a remedy or an alleviation for every infirmity incident to our fallen nature; but so much has the fashion of the times increased the use of foreign drugs, that it is now a question whether medicine be most beneficial or injurious to mankind. It is not the use, when guided by integrity, but the abuse of them, which proves a curse upon posterity; for the laws of physic are agreeable to the laws of Nature; its design is to preserve the body in health, to defend it from disease, to strengthen the weak, and to raise the dejected. According to the will of Providence, it is so ordained, for some wise purpose hitherto unknown to us, yet every day's experience proves to us that all creatures that live are liable to mischance, and that *"sickness and disease, which is painful to the body, may be profitable to the soul; it is the mother of modesty, that, while in the full career of worldly pomp and pride, kindly pulls us by the ear to bring us to a proper sense of our duty, and examine our substance whereof we are made, that millions of strange shadows on us tend."*

A man in humble life, blessed with a mode rate portion of common sense and honest intentions, assisted by medical reading, and directed by the simple dictates of Nature, is frequently more successful than many regular practitioners, who are so intent upon dosing their patient, that they often play with a disease, until in reality, they cannot cure it. This, without meaning any disrespect to the honest practitioner, I regret to say, I have often witnessed. Two ladies, in particular, who have kindly allowed me to refer to them, the one had been confined for five months to her room, and the other eleven months, under professional men. The first was perfectly restored in six, and the other in nine days, by taking my simple remedies, and have since remained in good health. About eighteen months ago, I was applied to by one of the members of the Central District Society in my neighbourhood, to attend two poor men, who were the greatest possible sufferers, and perfectly helpless. One had been so seven months, and the other nine; both were re stored to perfect health in eleven days. These cures I performed gratuitously, and felt amply repaid by knowing that I had restored two poor fellow-creatures to their distressed families; but the Society before-named voted me a remuneration for these cures. I could mention many similar cases, but have selected these particularly, as their truth can be easily ascertained. The satisfaction resulting from a sense of doing good to my fellow-creatures repays me for the jeers of self-exalted and ambitious men; for I am well aware that he who stands forward to promote a reform in any particular profession, must excite enmity, and draw on himself the clamour of interested individuals, who would wish to keep medicine clothed in a mystic garb, instead of being put upon a level with the plainest understanding, and rendered as obvious and familiar to us as the food we eat. - Vide Dr. Morrison's treatise of *"Medicine no Mystery."* Dr. Madden says, *"I disclaim all theories in a science like that of medicine. Where there are no general rules, there can be no unerring and universal principles."*

The brute creation possess discrimination in a surprising degree. Watch a dog when he is sick, and he will search for the *quich-grass*; if costive, he will choose some leaf of any of the *docks*. Wound a toad, and it is said he will travel until he finds some ground-sel or dandelion; when found, he will chew the herb until it becomes a salve, with which he will anoint his wounds, and cure them. Again, an ancient writer says, *"If you wound the eyes of young swallows, when in their nest, the old ones will again recover their sight with the herb of celandine; but,"* he adds, *"as it can answer no good purpose to torture helpless, unoffending creatures, I entreat my readers not to try such cruel and wicked experiments."*

Botanic medicine is yet in its infancy; and though a natural study has been banished from society, for unnatural drugs, my ambition will be satisfied if I have discovered one of its new rays.

It is expected in the medical profession, that when one of their members discovers a new mode of cure, he is to give up the secret to the faculty in general. If he refuses, they call him a *quack*, as in the case of Dr. James, with his powders, and many others before and after him. What encouragement is there for any man, under this system, to study for himself any new mode of cure, when this arbitrary custom would enable the stupid and indolent drone of the profession (for many there are) to participate in the profits of the ingenious discoverer? Many have lived, whose abilities would have proved an ornament to society, but whose study and acquirements were rendered entirely useless to them, because the present method prevents enter prize, and obliges them to proceed in one beaten path. But Abernethy said, in one of his lectures, *"he hoped he should live to see the day when this prejudice would be re moved."*

To the liberal part of the community, I might urge the sacrifices I have made, both of property and time, in conducting a course of experiments wholly unknown in the usual course of medical practice; and I trust that my opinion of the cause and treatment of Gout, &c. will be found stated in so plain a manner as to be easily understood; for when a professionally educated man, who has acquired his knowledge from others, and from his books, sits down to write, he is very apt to overlook the connection between scientific and common truths; he begins his treatise, not by a reference to something understood by every one, but imperceptible to all but those who have had a college education equal to his own. When a self- taught and self- educated man, as I am, attempts to explain to others what he himself has learned, he is less likely to fall into this error; having had no masters to supply the deficiencies of his own education, and this being such as common observation teaches every man, hereby there springs a method and style of address in every respect suited to general readers. He knows from his own experience what difficulties such readers have to contend with, and is the better qualified to guard against them; stating facts in common and simple language - avoiding all those figures and incomprehensible modes of expression in which the best writers have so much abounded; for, in physic, no figure of speech should be used, the use of which carries the mind from the things to be described; though they may amuse the collegian, yet they give only a confused notion to the many, without adding to the true knowledge of the cause or cure of disease.

I will here give my readers two specimens of this mystification. I ask, what opinion you can form in your own mind, from Dr. Fuller's explanation of the operation of hysterics? He says *"This and other foetid medicines take off hysteric fits, by handling the spirits roughly, and driving and dispersing them; for when they grow mutinous, and unequally dispersed, running in tumultuous clouds in some places, and leaving others ungarrisoned, and so either intermit their duty within the precincts of the brain or precordia, or else do it perversely, then the best course is to send such a stern remedy among them, as may use severe discipline, and lash and scourge them until they are glad to leave their disorders, and run to their proper post, and fall to their charge again!"* I will treat my readers with another dose from the celebrated Dr. Salmon, who says, "Fermentation is a certain manifestation of life, fitting it for a resuscitation, and without which it would remain captive, within the bonds or chains of death; or it is the breaking of the bonds of corruption and putrefaction by the power of life, assisted by the homogene matter and principle already freed."

Now I am bold to say, that in this little work I have stated, in about three lines which cannot be misunderstood, the meaning (if there is any) of all this long rigmarole of absurdities. Would not the sense have been better understood had they used only *these* six words, which I had written long before I read the above quotation: *"Motion is the expression of life."* On reflection, I am truly happy that I had not a medical college education, which might have so bothered my brains, that the small share of common sense which Nature has given me, might have been lost in confusion, and rendered useless to me and every one else.

The following are the opposite opinions of scientific men on the cause and cure of that complaint which I profess to understand, viz. Gout. Some suppose this disease is occasioned by an alkaline salt, and must be cured by an acid; while others have been of a directly contrary opinion, even blaming acids and advising alkalies.

Now my own opinion is that both of these theories are wrong. *"It is not for me to adjust such grave disputes"*, therefore I consulted my old friend Dr. Common Sense, who told me, even without fee or reward, that if Nature's operations be in any way retarded, an accumulation of oily matter in the blood immediately commences, which causes, more or less, swellings all over the body, as well in the dropsy, as in the gout. Now my treatment stirs up a fresh fermentation in the body, by means of which the sinking, and almost dying spirits become roused; the blood, recovering its due mixture, becomes released from coagulation and putrefaction; Nature makes a brisk effort, and expels the deleterious matter. My treatment for Gout, &c. is in conformmity with the operations of Nature, and by very simple means I purify the whole mass of blood of those unhealthy fluids, which if repelled, or allowed to remain, will bring on disease in some other form. Indeed a more powerful evidence of the origin of disease being attributable to the state of the fluids cannot be offered than the *Gout*; this disease will remove its position many times in one day - solids cannot thus change about; this therefore clearly proves, as I have before stated, that it is the accumulation of an acrid matter, shifting about in the circulating fluids, sometimes depositing itself in the joints, bringing on those calcareous substances, denominated chalk stones. Now, to prevent this there are two things especially to be done: first, the sizy concretions must be so dissolved that the blood may easily be returned into the veins again; secondly, the fibres must, by oily external applications, be made more limp and supple. This being accomplished, the continual motion of the blood acting on the fibres will recover their natural state, the congested humours become re-absorbed, and of course the distemper expelled.

Having spoken of humours in parts of my little work, I ought to acquaint my readers what I mean by the term. There are four in number, viz. blood, phlegm, choler, and melancholy. *First,* blood is in its nature uncorrupted, therefore hot, gummy, and sweet in taste; but society having, for generations past, got into an artificial and luxurious way of living, different from what Nature first intended, is the reason why so much medicine is required to heck those gross humours which such excess of diet always generates.

> "But when we have stuffed
> These pipes and these conveyances of our blood
> With wine and feeding, we have suppler souls
> Than in our priest-like fast."

> "Give me excess of it, that surfeiting,
> The appetite may sicken, and so die."
>   SHAKSPEARE.

> The first physicians by debauch were made,
> Excess began, and Sloth sustains the trade.
> By work our long-lived fathers earned their food,
> Toil strung the nerves, and purified the blood.
> But we their sons - a pampered race of men,
> Are dwindled down to three-score years and ten;
> Better to hunt in fields for health unbought,
> Than fee the doctor for a nauseous draught;
> The wise for cure on exercise depend,
> God never made his work for man to mend.
>   DRYDEN.

Secondly, phlegm is cold and moist, and either sweet or without taste at all. *Thirdly,* the choleric humour is hot and dry, and very bitter in taste. *Fourthly,* the melancholy humour is cold and dry, and in taste very sour. Blood may be compared to air; phlegm to water; choler to fire; and melancholy to earth. All the humours are mixed through the whole of the body, and I account for the different constitutions and dispositions of men but by the fact, that these humours in their several qualities abound more in one individual than in another. I consider the body as a system of tubes and glands, or, to use a more homely phrase, a bundle of pipes and strainers, fitted to one another after so wonderful a manner as to make a proper engine for the soul to work with. This description not only comprehends the bowels, bones, tendons, veins, nerves, and arteries, but every muscle, and every ligament, which is a composition of fibres, that are so many imperceptible tubes or pipes interwoven on all sides with invisible glands or strainers.

This general idea of a human body, without considering it in its niceties of anatomy, shews us how absolutely necessary labour is for the right preservation of it. There must be frequent agitations, to mix, digest, and separate the juices contained in it, as well as to clear and cleanse that infinitude of pipes and strainers of which it is composed, and to give their solids a more firm and lasting tone. Labour or exercise ferments the humours, casts them into their proper channels, throws off redundancies, and helps nature in those secret distributions, without which the body cannot subsist in its vigour, nor the soul act with cheerfulness. I might here mention the effects which this has upon all the faculties of the mind; keeping the understanding clear, the imagination untroubled, and refining those spirits that are necessary for the proper exertion of our intellectual faculties, under the present laws of union between soul and body. It is to a neglect in this particular that we must ascribe the spleen, which is so frequent in men of studious and sedentary habits, as well as the vapours to which those of the other sex are so often subject. Had not exercise been absolutely necessary for our well-being, Nature would not have so adapted the human frame for it, giving such an activity to the limbs, and such a pliancy to every part, as necessarily produce those compressions, extensions, contortions, dilatations, and all other kinds of motions necessary for the preservation of such a system of tubes and glands as has been before mentioned.

This law of Nature has been acknowledged by the highest authority, namely, the Bible; in the book of Ecclesiasticus it is said: *"All things are double one against another, and he hath made nothing imperfect; one thing establisheth the good of another."* Read another truth of the same book: *"Nothing has been created in vain."* Now, while those humours possess their natural qualities, and their just proportions, so long they are wholesome and good; but when they become disordered and corrupted for want of proper diet, medicine, or exercise, then they are unwholesome, and no longer to be denominated by their proper name, but may be properly called melancholy blood, diseased phlegm, fever, burnt choler, and fretting melancholy. From these causes, in my opinion, proceed every kind of disease, call it by what name you may. These humours are like branches of a tree, from which spring other humours, either to do them service or an injury, as the case may be, by their action on the three natural powers, *viz.* the power animal, the power natural, and the power vital. The power animal is dependent on the brain, which gives feeling and motion to all parts of the body; the power vital, is a virtue belonging only to the heart, which gives life and spirit to the whole body by means of the arteries; the power natural, belonging to the digestive organs, which give nourishment to the body. The power natural has four other particulars, *viz.* attractive, which draws nutriment from the food to sustain the body; the retentive, by which it retains and keeps the food received; the digestive, which concocts and digests the same; and lastly, the expulsive, by which is thrown off the excrementitious and superfluous parts of the food. These actions must be perfect, according to the rules of Nature, for a man to enjoy good health, to secure which, I would recommend proper diet, air, and exercise. It requires very little study to understand the three following humours, and then to know a quick and safe remedy. Say, if the blood is over heated, use the herb called red centaury in an infusion; if choler, use the yellow centaury herb; if of phlegm, the white of the same sort will be found beneficial. I think it would be well if this knowledge were a part of the education of every school-boy; but this not being the custom of the present day, is the fault of society (upon whom also falls the punishment thereof), and not the fault of Nature, for she from time to time makes man a present of varieties, both useful and agreeable; but the miseries accumulated by mankind, pass from huts to palaces, from ages past to ages yet to come; and the two epidemic plagues, which one after the other have visited our shores for the last three years, and still remain with us to this moment, cry with a loud and fearful voice in the ears of every man, Study Nature's laws in all her ways, and oppress not the miserable. Others as well as myself must have discovered that additional diseases are continually arising, and showing themselves, if possible, in a more fatal point of view. This is what was to be expected. Disease can only be subdued in one way, by eradicating it; but it cannot be stifled; if this is attempted, it shews itself in another form and quarter. The nation will, ere long, it is to be hoped, turn its thoughts to the knowledge of what true health, and the means of attaining it, consists in; it will be found much more profitable than in submitting to the present jobbing in disease, when they have the remedy in their own hands:

"What need we have any friends if we should never have need of them? We are all born to do benefits: and what better or properer can we call our own than the riches of our friends?" - SHAKSPEARE

Then let our friends the Government look to this. Shakspeare must have had some such thoughts when, in speaking of a government, he says,

"There is a sickness
Which puts some of us in distemper, but
I cannot name the disease, and it is caught
Of you that yet are well."

Cholera is said to arise from impurity of the air: in my opinion, there would not be an un wholesome spot on the face of the earth if man had not made it so; no air is unwholesome but where there is corruption. The purple fever, the dysentery, the small-pox, the measles, so common in our villages when the season has been warm proceed for the most part from the puddles of the village, in which leaves of many of the most useful plants are left to putrify; and many of our city distempers arise from dunghills, and from the burial of the dead in our closely inhabited church- yards. The corruption of the air is a subject which concerns every man; and I would suggest the same means for remedying it as I do for all diseases: first, remove the cause, and the effects will follow.

It cannot be denied by any man of the least observing mind, but that the weather or air have great effect on the earth, animals, vegetables, and also the human body, according to that description of humour which every man and herb more or less abounds in. Can we be surprised at this, when we see it act on stone and brick walls, on iron, copper, tin, in fact on every thing on the face of the earth! Hippocrates affirms: *"The air is the cause of the most terrible distempers and epidemic diseases, by which mortals are hurried into the other world, and which arises from no other cause than the malignity of the air; for the circulation of the blood bears a proportion to the state of the air, and health bears a direct proportion to the state of the blood. The manner in which this seems to be performed is by refraction, compression, and direction of motion on this or that humour."*

Great care should be taken in thickly populated neighbourhoods to prevent the bodies and offal of dead animals from being thrown into their laystals. Who can conceive the danger of drinking the *stinking Thames water,* such as is found in part of the Thames between Greenwich and Twickenham, contaminated by the filth it receives from a city containing nearly two millions of people! The drainings of laystals, thousands of stables and slaughter-houses, gas-works, factories - all this filthy mixture is kept in a fermented state by the ebbing and flowing of the tide, which prevents its being carried away, and in this state it is conveyed to the cisterns; which, when blended with our food in the stomach, causes another fermentation to commence, preventing digestion, and causing every kind of inflammatory disease; and, the knowledge that this evil still exists, and in proportion to the increase of population, becoming worse, must be revolting to our nature, and to every reflecting mind. Hoffman tells us, that putrid waters - *"will not only corrupt the air, but are likewise capable of producing scrofulous tumours, putrid diseases, and all kind of fevers."* The water companies should be compelled to bring their water (which may be easily done) from above where the tide ceases to flow. I am convinced that thousands would have suffered much less bodily pain than they have done, or even do now, if this had been insisted on years ago. To suppose that so much disease can arise, which we every day see increasing, without such causes producing them, would be a libel on the Author of Nature. Then to remove this nuisance would be acting on one of those common laws of universal justice, whose precept enjoins on us to consider all men as brethren, and to study their comfort and interest equally with our own. This is the purpose for which we have been born; however others may argue that self preservation is the first law of nature, this selfish opinion will not harmonize with her laws, for does not nature allow man almost exclusively to enjoy a long period of life, be cause even in old age he may be useful to his fellow-creature?

On the Use of Vapour Baths in the Treatment of Gout.

In my former work I stated, I had invented an apparatus for giving a medicated bath in bed at the patient's own home. My patients, both from town and country, soon became so numerous, that I was under the necessity of going to a heavy expense in erecting baths, and arranging that the steam may be conveyed to every part of my house, which is very extensive, My mode of giving baths is very different from any other, I believe, in the metropolis. I never suffer patients to go out after having taken them, but they are immediately put into a warm bed; and in very bad cases I afterwards give them a medicated hot-air bath, to keep up the perspiration. As I attend every gentleman's bath myself, (Mrs. Tilke attending the ladies,) I cannot give them by day; therefore those patients who do not reside in my house, come from seven to eleven in the evening, and remain all night. My number of resident patients is limited to six, being as many as I can do my duty by; and of the great number of patients I have had, there is not one but I can with pride refer to. I do consider these baths the greatest improvement in administering vegetable matter to the stomach and lungs ever invented. Their power in removing spasms I have proved to be very great; this alone would prove a great blessing to mankind.

One of the principal agents I employ for the removal of the Gout, is an ointment which I prepare for the purpose, which is to be applied by way of friction, for the purpose of promoting a free discharge of perspirable matter, and which, at the same time, conveys its specific action to the parts affected by means of the nerves and absorbent vessels. The astonishing efficacy of this ointment, in relieving almost immediately the most inveterate attacks of gout, as well as rheumatism, lumbago, and cramp, is proved by the attestation of numerous highly respectable individuals, who have been cured by it, and who are most anxious to give every information as to its virtues, action, safety, and certainty.

Another agent in aid of the cure of this distressing malady consists in paying proper attention, at the same time, to the digestive organs, which will be effected by taking the pills prepared by me for this purpose, independently of a certain influence they possess over the whole system, necessary to assist the action of the ointment before alluded to: and as much depends on a proper condition of the lower bowels, or that portion of the bowels called the rectum and the colon, it is frequently advisable to stimulate them by the use of injections, or simple lavements of warm water, which is best effected by perhaps one of the most simple, and at the same time one of the most effective apparatus ever shewn to the public, which I keep and sell for that purpose.

The medicated vapour-baths which I apply to the patient, enables me to medicate the system by the agency of the lungs, whereby the blood partakes of all the properties of the herbs without inconvenience to the digestive organs; and this latter plan of treatment I frequently find of the utmost benefit in my practice; as many persons apply to me whose constitutions are so overcharged with medicine, such as colchicum and other pernicious and poisonous ingredients, that it is with difficulty I can at first get my ointment to act, unless assisted by this plan of carrying my remedy to the seat of the disease. But by the application of the ointment alone, I have, in most cases, been enabled to effect a speedy cure; in no case, however difficult, or of very long standing, wherein I have been compelled to call in my whole battery of agents or remedies, have I ever been defeated; the more difficult the case, the more astonishing and wonderful appear the result. In fact, in no instance within my own observation, have my plans failed in effecting a perfect cure.

Strict attention to the purity of person cannot be too much recommended; as the matter thrown out by perspiration, if permitted to accumulate on the surface of the skin, closes the pores, and occasions disorders that might be prevented by occasionally taking a steam-bath, as the circulation is brought from the centre to the surface of the body, and the pores are freed from foulness by the heat and expulsive power of the herbs, which tends as well to alleviate any local irritation, and thereby to produce sleep. By this easy means of administering vegetable medicine, no vessel is strained; all the secretions are performed with great facility, as the internal organs open and discharge themselves when perspiration takes place. I have proved to many of my scientific patients, men whom I can refer to, that by a proper selection of herbs, and being acquainted with their great power, producing calmness, refreshment, emollient, diluting, gently opening, diuretic, causing a great desire for food; these baths, in fact, accomplish as much means in one hour, as taking medicine by the mouth will do in ten. Then how necessary must this be in all fevers! *"A crisis,"* says a learned author, *"is the actual discharge of morbid matter, whether by the bowels or skin, brought on by the powers of nature, or the aid of medicine."* There the bath is the aid at once, for by its effects the discharge may be brought on at pleasure. *Scantorius* found, by experiments, that the excretions made by the human body in a given time were commonly in the following proportions: by stool, four; urine, sixteen; and through the pores of the body, forty. This will have the same effect on the bodies of those without any feverish disease; such as come under the description of dropsy, or a general swelling or puffing of the body, or only that of the limbs. Scrofula, all scorbutic complaints, distension of the stomach, scarcity of urine, leprosy, and many other complaints, must be benefited by the above treatment. The aged of both sexes will find the use of this bath prevent the fibres from becoming rigid, by giving free circulation, which must contribute to give them a long and comfortable life, as the great warmth diminishes and softens the tension of the solids, which cause the secretions to be mild and easy; for no person can enjoy an easy and good state of health, where perspiration is not properly promoted; and that cannot possibly be the case where exercise is neglected, for without exercise, the offensive matter cannot be thrown off; it must then be retained in the body, vitiating the humours, often producing fevers, head-aches, lumbago, pains of the stomach, gout, rheumatism, indigestion, and many other evils, that bring *grist* to the doctor's *mill.* Now' to those who cannot possibly take exercise, the bath is the only substitute for it; for I am of opinion, when these matters are attended to, it is impossible for an *hepatic* disease to exist; but when the pores of the skin are closed, when the orifices of the surface that are by nature intended to discharge the superfluities of the body become closed, then is the liver over-clogged with juices that are repelled from the surface. Experience with my baths, on those sent to me by the profession for the liver complaint, have shown me these effects; but reason and reflexion first pointed out to me the cause. That a connexion exists between the skin and all the internal organs which act in sympathy with the liver, the habitual drunkard gives us one proof; for the skin of his face becomes florid and turgid with blood, and the nose particularly is often covered with eruptions, even to deformity: showing, or rather say convincing us, that there are some irregularities in the functions of his liver, which leaves other signs, such as a *leaden colour of the skin, deadness of the eye, emasciation, depression of spirits, and diminution of muscular power.* I have also found the use of baths, medicinally conducted, and persisted in for a proper time, will effect most extraordinary cures in the dropsy. It is of consequence to be able to distinguish this complaint from another which bears some likeness to it, as it regards some effects that females at the turn of life experience, when an oily, glutinous humour accumulates instead of water. This I know to be contrary to the general opinion, *but this is mine*; and I consider practical results as outweighing theoretical conclusions; to the former alone I appeal. It was reasoning on the wonderful works of nature, and some accidental occurrences, that first convinced me how necessary it was to apply different herbs in the bath, &c. to remove those two similar causes that produce but one effect; accordingly I reduced my views to practice, and the result has been such as to corroborate them in every point of view. Diet and regimen are very important branches of the treatment of those two complaints, as well as gout, as they not only assist in removing the more urgent symptoms, but are also the best means of preventing the returns of attack. Liquors of all kinds that are not well fermented, are pernicious for the gout, rheumatism, and dropsy; as the narcotic principle they contain renders them objectionable for this reason, it induces a sluggishness of the veins, which prevents them from transmitting the blood from the different organs with the same quickness as it is propelled into them by the arteries. Hence we find, in attacks of gout, the limbs swell, and the blood curdles and is so thick it cannot pass through the veins.

"This is, as I take it, a kind of lethargy, a kind of sleeping in the blood; it hath its origin from much grief, from study and perturbation in the brain. I have read the cause of it in Galen." - SHAKSPEARE.

This subject has been one of the most important of my studies; and I must confess I have had *"ten thousand thoughts that died in thinking"* on that power which regulates the circulation of the blood. This is the grand point every man who pretends to the study of medicine ought to steer for. I hope ere long the profession will be convinced of this fact.

To those who suffer with the gout, and have not the assistance of either the medicated or vapour baths, the following directions will be found sufficient, and with perseverance, a cure is certain. Apply the ointment freely to the parts affected (and across the chest and loins, the real seat of the disease, although pains may be experienced in other parts of the body and limbs); let the ointment be rubbed in till pimples make their appearance, which is a sure symptom of the CAUSE of the disease being gradually removed from the region of the liver and kidneys, and with a judicious use of the prepared pills, which I recommend to be taken at the same time, the EFFECTS also will speedily vanish. The rubbing should be continued with the hand for at least twenty minutes once a day, and not less than half a pot used each time (for much depends upon its being sufficiently rubbed in); immediately afterwards the parts to be covered with wadding and flannel, by which means a comfortable warmth is kept up, thereby greatly facilitating the cure. There are at the same time the following precautions proper to be attended to by the patient; *viz.* 1st. On commencing with the ointment, to be particular in attending to the bowels. 2dly. To be resolute in the rubbing, being certain that temporary pain will be succeeded by a positive cure. And 3dly, That in most cases it is preferable that the patient do not leave the bed while using this very harmless ointment, as the perspiration should be promoted, not checked.

It is well known there are many species of gout, and according to the constitution the ointment has different effects; with some it promotes the swelling, but causes almost instant ease, and performs an immediate cure; while with others it reduces the swelling and inflammation, but gives pain for two or three days, at the end of which time a few small pimples will appear, which is a good symptom. At any future time, should the patient feel the least return of the complaint, by immediately fomenting the part with hot water, and having recourse to the ointment, it will draw off the attack in a few hours. Soaking the feet, and rubbing in a little ointment once a week, and taking one pill about every second or third day, will keep the blood in a good state, and prevent any future attack.

The following gentlemen have supplied their names for the purpose of affording every explanation as to the efficacy of the ointment, as experienced by themselves and friends:

Mr. Coleman, 6, Westmoreland Street, Mary-le-bone.
Mr. Harrison, No. 1, Little Woodstock Street.
Mr. Winter, 69, East Street, Manchester Square.
Mr. Sweetland, corner of John Street and Howland Street, Fitzroy Square.

Mr. Huntley, 294, Regent Street; and 281, Oxford Street.
Mr. Hutchins, St. Luke's Head, King Street, Park Street.
Mr. Gregory, 100, Kingsland Road.
Mr. Hasystey, Coal-Harbour Street, Hackney Road.
Mr. Beard, 14, James Place, Marlbro ' Road, Chelsea.
Mr. Elsmore, 27, High Street.
Mr. Crawley, 22, Beaumont Street.
Mr. Etheridge, Featherstone Buildings, Limehouse.
J. Pope, Esq., Gray's Buildings, Ball's Pond, Islington.
Mr. Paull, 10, Great Chesterfield Street.
Mr. Keeble, 1, High Street.
Mr. Gibbins, 13, High Street.
R. Bennet, Esq., 11, William Street, Hampstead Road.
William Hubble, Esq., York Terrace, Regent's Park.
Mr. Simmons, 3, Grove Terrace, Regent's Park.
Mr. King, Charles Street, Manchester Square.
Mr. Turner, near Union Hall, Borough.
Mr. Hodges, Lord Somers' Arms, Somers Town.
Mr. Foster, 43, East Street.

At the suggestion of many of my patients, particularly those living in the country, whom I have supplied with baths, I now give notice, that I will furnish families with my little steam apparatus, which may be used in bed, or it will act out of bed under a canopy, and herbs prepared for the occasion according to the nature of the complaint. This little useful bath ought to be kept in every house, for by its timely application, many a long and serious illness might be prevented; as with three or four ounces of spirits of wine, one quart of boiling water, and the prepared herbs, in ten minutes the heat will be got as high as 130 degrees.

TILKE'S *improved Hot-air Bath and Bed Warmer.*

This little apparatus, with one ounce of spirits of wine, will burn one hour, and warm the bed from 110 to 120 degrees; and by putting a piece of camphor on the wire, the patient may have a camphorated bath for about three-pence. This is a very excellent companion in a carriage in cold damp weather, or to persons living alone, as there is no assistance wanting, and on getting into bed, they may be moved to any part, as there is no danger, being made on the principle of Sir Humphrey Davy's lamp. Price £1.5s. to £1. 10s.

My ointment may be used with perfect safety on the most tender infant for the Spasms; and for adults, in all cases of Pleuresy, Cholera Morbus, Sore Throats, Sprains, &c. In fact, for almost every complaint at tended with pain, it will give immediate relief. Sold in Pots (duty included) at 4s. 6d. and 2s. 9d. each. Pills, ls. 1d. per box; and 2s. 9d. per bottle.

By S. W. Tilke, No. 8, Thayer Street, Manchester Square.

ON DIET.

I have said little on diet in these pages; indeed, no positive rule can be laid down. All men, by exercising the ability God has given them, can well judge for themselves. I shall give a few simple hints while at meals; and first, I shall state what Mr. Jukes says in his excellent little work.

"It is impossible to lay down a definite system of diet; it is a question involved in much perplexity, and has even been a subject for controversial writers. An organ like the stomach, which has been known to digest brass buttons, pins, and even clasp knives; while others, on the contrary, have suffered the most serious inconvenience by the mere smell or reception of a trifling quantity of food apparently of the most simple kind." — Dr. Gall could never partake of mutton, dressed, in whatever manner, with out suffering irritation in his stomach to a most distressing degree, proving, that in some constitutions the mildest food may be the most injurious. Veal, ham, puddings, and pies, act similarly with myself. I have given my opinion on this cause in my explanation of the four humours in another part of this work.

> "Some men there are, love not a gaping pig;
> Some, that are mad, if they behold a cat;
> And others, when the bag-pipe sings,
> Cannot contain themselves; for affection
> Masterly passion, sways it to the mood
> Of what it likes, or loaths:
> As there is no firm reason to be rendered,
> So I can give no reason, nor I will not."
> SHAKSPEARE.

It appears so inconsistent in the execution of its functions as almost to defy any attempt at prescribed rules for diet. Mr. Jukes says, *"Persons who have arrived at maturity are, or ought to be, the best judges of the quantity of food the stomach will contain and digest easily. A knowledge that requires neither learning or science, yet there are times when this organ requires more than usual humouring, in consequence of its great disposition to sympathize with every other part of the body. We should regulate our system of diet in conformity with our age, habits, infirmities, and avocations; our stomachs naturally differ from each other quite as much as one man's countenance differs from another; for it would be worse than nonsense to suppose that the stomach of the abstemious, and that of the drunkard, are alike."* In speaking of the latter, he says, *"Drunkenness lowers man beneath the brute; it weakens the digestive organs, impairs the memory."* Another author has said, *"Drunkenness expels reason, drowns the memory, defaces beauty, diminishes strength, inflames the blood* (which causes gout), *causes external and incurable wounds, is a witch to the senses, a devil to the soul, a thief to the purse, the beggar's companion, the wife's woe, and the children's sorrow; makes a strong man weak, and a wise man a fool - for he is a self-murderer who drinks to others' good health, and robs himself of his own."* I have copied this as being in perfect unison with my own opinion although I could not have found words equally strong; for I do feel that the two greatest curses that ever fell on this country or any other are the sale of ardent spirits, and the use of mercury as medicine. Dr. Price tells us, that only one in a hundred of such persons lives to be eighty years of age, while the Quakers average one in ten. There cannot be a more powerful argument used to support the practice of temperance, which keeps the pulsation at the regular temperature, say, when in health, about eighty beats to a minute; but if by excess of eating or drinking, or other cause, a person inflames the blood, raising the pulse from 140 to that of 160, he must be wearing out nature's machine in one half of its time. Those persons from habit at last are obliged to continue the *spur* of excitement to keep them to a certain *focus*, until nature gives way. This is a class of men I pity above all others, seeing that of all miserable lives this must be the most wretched. I shall now close these remarks with the following hint: First, *consult your stomach,* to find out what it will digest and what it will not; and I by no means advise any persons to drink fermenting liquors while at meals, as it sets the stomach fermenting instead of digesting. My readers will find a diet drink for meals at the end of this book; simple, easy to make, very cheap, and a very great assistant to the stomach which is weak in its digestive powers.

ON PLANTS AND FLOWERS.

"All arts and sciences are more or less encumbered with vulgar errors and prejudices, which avarice and ignorance have sufficient influence to preserve by help of mysterious, undefinable, and not seldom unintelligible technical terms or nicknames which serve only to shroud it in almost impenetrable obscurity; and so fond are the professors of an art of keeping up all the pomp, circumstance, and mystery of it, that one might fairly suppose those who have had the courage and perseverance to overcome these obstacles, and penetrate the veil of science, were delighted with placing difficulties in the way of those who may attempt to follow them, on purpose to deter them from the pursuit; and that they cannot bear that others should climb the hill of knowledge by an easier road than they themselves had; and that as their predecessors supported themselves by serving out with a sparing hand, the information they so hardly obtained, they find it convenient to follow their example, and willing to do as they have been done by, leave and bequeath the inheritance undiminished to those who may succeed them." - Dr. KITCHENER.

As regards the power of different herbs variously used, I will point out the following seeming paradoxes, hitherto unaccounted for. The herb called crow-fig, or *nux vomica,* given to some descriptions of dogs, will instantly deprive them of nervous energy, and in five minutes destroy life, while the same herb may be given to other dogs without their being affected by it. The root alkanet (or, as the Profession call it, *radix anchusa),* is in no degree hurtful to man; is is even beneficial to children made into an infusion, to drive out the small-pox or measles; yet this same herb will destroy either dog or cat. My remedy for Rheumatism acts precisely the same both on man and dog; although there is this difference in the complaint (as justly observed by a very ingenious writer), that rheumatism in the dog never exists without affecting the bowels. The powder of mistletoe, which grows on the hazel tree, is a cure for most persons troubled with fits, if about four drachms a day be taken in holy thistle tea; yet with dogs and horses it has no effect. Again, if a man places a small portion of the herb purslain under his tongue, it will quench thirst; but if a dog take it, the instant he has his liberty he will fly to the first water he can reach, be it ever so impure, to slake his intolerable thirst; there is even reason to believe that a dog in a rabid state would be compelled to drink after chewing it. In another part of my little work will be found a further enumeration of the peculiar properties of many herbs and roots, kindly bestowed upon us by a beneficent Providence, but which, I fear, are altogether undervalued at the present day.

Will it be contended that vegetable productions, such as I have described, (and, be it observed, there are thousands possessing equally astonishing properties), were meant by our all-powerful Creator, to lie "cumbering the ground," totally unregarded? or, rather, were they not all supplied each for some specific and useful purpose? Let our modern Pharmacopoeias contain even but a moderate list of those useful medicines to be found in almost every field and valley, and less anxiety be shewn in digging from the bowels of the earth minerals, which in many cases are but sorry substitutes for what is to be found on the surface: we may then calculate upon more certain and less dilatory progress in the curative art.

The careful searcher after botanical knowledge will find in the works of many of our early authors most invaluable information on the medicinal properties of herbs. One of our sage writers wittily remarks, in his peculiarly quaint manner, *"Why do men die, while sage in garden grows?"* I can bear testimony to the virtues of this much-neglected herb, useful in many cases, and injurious in none. The writings of Dr. Thornton may be read with great advantage by the student; and a paper by Dr. Jackson, inserted in the Medical and Physical Journal for February 1810, on his discovery and trials of the virtues of 'Eyebright', will afford one specimen of what yet remains to be done in the botanical world, where discoveries may be made every step we take, in whatever path we tread.

It may not, perhaps, be out of place to state here, that my own natural inclination has, from early childhood, been led to the study of medicine. This fondness for the pursuit, although in some degree inherited from my father (who was clever, in the veterinary art,) met with no encouragement from my parents; and although a medical gentleman (Mr. Hodges, still living at Sidmouth, Devon) offered, when I was but nine years of age, to take me entirely under his tuition, still I was consigned to another pursuit. But the one favourite study haunted my mind during anxious days and sleepless nights, brooding over the yet untried inventions of my own, and storing my mind with the many valuable truths, to be found by an attentive reader, in writers on botanical medicine. I need hardly say, that I did not arrive at my present limited knowledge of medicine but by degrees. My first cures were in the more simple complaints to which human nature is liable. These, and the cure of Ring-worm (which I have performed many years), and my more recent discovery of a cure for the Gout, have now for above four years placed me very prominently before the Public eye. And I now most solemnly state, that in no case have I ever heard of injurious effects from the modes of cure, but that I have received the thanks and blessings of my patients beyond my most sanguine expectations.

Many of our most useful plants we undervalue because they are common and everywhere to be found. I will give a case in proof. About two years since a medical gentleman in great practice, residing a few miles from town, brought to me his only daughter, a most accomplished young lady, afflicted with a disease considered, as he himself said, incurable. I found him a candid and sensible man: he told me who and what he was, and admitted that for three years he had had the first advice in London, together with his own assistance, without success. He said, *"I suppose you think it strange that I should apply to you, and I assure you I had at first a struggle with my own feelings; but having been a witness of a cure you performed on the daughter of a professional man, I am sure you can cure mine: here, Sir, is a cheque for a sum of money, and when cured you shall receive another to the same amount."* I told him it was not a case I professed to understand, and I wished to confine myself to Gout and the cure of Ring-worm only; but as he had behaved so handsomely, and as it always gave me pleasure to communicate to and aid others with the knowledge of my own discoveries, I would assist him. Judge of his surprise when I told him how to prepare duckmeat, chickweed, and groundsil. *"Why,"* says he, *"I have a pond at the back of my house with abundance of duckmeat, and the other two grow in my garden!"* Here was a college-educated man using useless drugs, procured hundreds and thousands of miles, when nature had planted the very remedy as it were at the threshold of his own door. The young lady only paid me three visits, and was cured in two months. So much for plants that are thought useless, because nature has been so kind as to make them common amongst us. Many of the most useful grow all the year round. I am only sorry that mankind do not study the utility of their qualities for health, nourishment, and pleasure. I would refer to the instinct of animals; watch them when feeding, and you will see them vary the choice of their pasture; their knowledge emanates from laws of a superior order, into which, while in this world, we shall never be able to penetrate; and if such knowledge elude our researches, we must consider it is for the general good of all beings on earth, especially that of man; for on examination we shall find nature raises the physical character of her works by collecting them around mankind. Every plant that grows in the corn-fields possesses virtues adapted to the maladies incidental to the condition of the labourer; for let him take whatever pains he may in sifting the grain and weeding his field, the two following plants are always found mixed with the standing corn, *viz.* the *poppy*, which is a safe cure for the pleurisy, eases pain, and procures sleep; stops hemorrhages and spitting of blood; and the *blue-bottle*, which is a diuretic, it softens and extends the fibres which compose the uririnary glands and channels to carry off the casual intrusion of particles too big to pass by the usual and common means.

I could much enlarge on these bounties of nature; but my patients will bear me out in the assertion that my present engagements will not admit of it; yet I hope to live to see the day in which I shall be enabled to satisfy mankind, that nature is the best contriver and compounder of her own productions: for those two simple plants the properties of which so well blend and work together for both to answer their important ends at once, I trust will serve as a good hint to those who only practise with the means which the art of man has contrived as a substitute for the works of nature. My readers perhaps may ask, why injurious and artificial substitutes should still remain in use in these enlightened days? My answer is, because following the beaten track contributes to the ease of the lazy, money making, college-bred doctors. *"Go to the ant, thou sluggard; consider her ways, and be made wise; which having no guide, overseer, or ruler, provideth her meat in the summer, and gathereth her food in the harvests."* Prov. iv. 6. Nature has composed her works in such a way as always to have novelty, in order to keep man, as well as beast, continually in exercise.

From this observation I would draw also this conclusion, that the Author of Nature intended to link mankind together by a union and interchange of thought for each others' benefit, the chain of which I fear is very much disjointed. Some persons may answer, *"this is only opinion"*: right; for where is the man who has become thoroughly acquainted with the endless views of nature? For *"to whom hath the root of wisdom been revealed, and who hath known her wise counsels?"* Ecclesiastes, chap. i . ver. 6.

> "We, ignorant of ourselves,
> Beg often our own harms, which the wise powers
> Deny us for our good: so find we profit,
> By losing of our prayers."
>   SHAKSPEARE,

But Nature assists those who study her works, and makes them wise, from the means she employs to accomplish the ends she purposes. This is one of the strongest proofs of a Divine Benevolence. Nature permits man only to know the end she has in view; it is on this she wishes his heart and mind to be fixed; she has no wish to make him ingenious and proud; her object is to render him virtuous, by which means he will also be happy, She is always ready to mitigate his difficulties and multiply his blessings. I am borne out in this opinion by an authority which will never deceive: (*Ecclesiasticus,* chap. iii. from the 17th to the 24th verse.) Were we to study the relation which many plants have to animals, we should discover the use of many of them. Nature has established among them individuals which are of different sexes; like to the animal creation. Many are found united in clusters, which show us the wish to live in each other's company; many have their likes and their dislikes, and will not grow or multiply near each other. Others, like hermits, are always to be found in a state of solitude. The male and female drake, although growing together, I have known to be as different in their virtues as light to dark. Mushrooms again present to us a multitude of contrasts, more so than any other production in our country. I have no doubt there are as many as fifty different species of them, all good when properly employed; in nature the simplest remedies produce the most useful effects, and in the early period of the world, when the art of medicine was practised more from motives of benevolence than gain, the world was less afflicted with disease. Very much depends upon the period and manner of collecting the herbs and roots intended for pharmaceutical purposes; yet very little attention is paid to this in the collection of what few medical herbs are used in this country. Their greatest favourites are gathered by the Moors in Africa, and the Indians in America, in *all seasons* of the year; they dry them carelessly in the sun
when the oils and other valuable medical properties are completely lost, it is not therefore at all surprising that, when brought to market, they fail in relieving the great mass of human suffering. There is a wide field open for investigation, and we shall find by close study, that the laws of life and health may be brought to a state of perfection far beyond the present conceptions of men. I would

advise the younger branches of the medical profession, who have not been conversant with studies of this kind, that they would put a better value upon such knowledge than heretofore, and not content themselves by serving an apprenticeship, or receiving a diploma; they should bear in mind that, to have a perfect insight into human nature, requires more study, insight, and perseverance, than is, according to the present practice, thought necessary. Every man has the power within himself of gaining this insight; he must shake off all prejudices against propositions deviating in any degree from the practice of the College of Physicians, and if he has but a moderate share of liberality, he will discover their error and pride without a pair of spectacles; and then it will be for him to form his own opinion whether it savours more of ignorance and folly than good sense and courtesy; he must examine into the *cause* of every thing, for he must be impressed with this simple and honest truth, that there can be no effect without a cause. He must bear in mind that health is *natural* to man, and that there is a cause when it is otherwise. The more he advances in this study, the more he will be satisfied that he is coming at the truth, and that he has heretofore been like a mariner without his compass. In this study they will immediately perceive that they ought to be very well acquainted with the virtues, faults, preparations, compositions, and proper doses of all vegetable medicine with which they practise. They ought to consider the regularity or irregularity of their patients, and then have the skill to judge for whom, for what, when, how much, and how often they are to administer to effect that change in the system, by purging, perspiration, or other evacuations.

To accomplish all this, a man had need to be rightly born and furnished by nature with a peculiar genius, and with a strong prevailing inclination for this study and practice; above all others, he must also be blessed with courage and activity, such as will bear him up and carry him through difficulties without on the one hand presumptuous rashness, or on the other, needless fear. I say, if a man is not by nature possessed of the above qualifications, all the study, all the practice, all the hammering into the brain, together with the best collection of books ever formed, can never make Nature's Physician, any more than good colours alone can make a fine painter, or that he should be made a jeweller whom Nature only intended for a blacksmith. I think Dr. Badham, in one of his recent lectures at Glasgow, must have been something of the same opinion, when he told his students: *"I have had,"* said he, *"many gentlemen in this class who have hovered about these smoky walls for seven or eight years, who have gone through six months' courses, and (not a few of them several times), in the ancient languages and mathematics, in LOGIC, in moral and experimental philosophy; in short, performed a complete course in the gowned classes before they put their hands upon the ark of medicine."* Now I would ask, must it not have been a torture to those poor young men to be compelled to be doctors, against Nature and their own inclinations? Had their natural abilities been studied, as it was the duty of their parents to have done, they might have been made good sailors, soldiers, wheelwrights, tailors, shoemakers, or taken up other honourable and respectable employments in life; but I would would wager St. Paul's Cathedral to an eggshell that they will never make good and useful doctors.

That the power of memory, reason, and the imagination, are bestowed in different portions to different men, may be known by every hour's experience.

> "These are begot in the ventricle of memory, nourished in the womb of *pia mater,*
> and delivered upon the mellowing of occasion: but the gift is good in those in whom it is acute."
> SHAKSPEARE.

We may observe that all the labours of education cannot overcome a natural dullness of capacity. High intellectual qualities may justly be called gifts, because they cannot be purchased by labour or wealth. It is not difficult to discover this mind and talent in a youth if they really exist; for I am of opinion that we have all our several parts assigned to us in this world, and those who have not a capacity for the liberal sciences, may upon examination, either by themselves or their friends, discover some talent of their own, useful in the pursuit of both public and private advantage. Many who have not genius for philosophy or polite learning, commonly enjoy, in a superior degree, common sense and courage, and possess a turn for study and usefulness sufficient to distinguish them in the more active scenes of life; for we cannot will of ourselves to be born wise, any more than to be born rich or poor; for God hath the appointment thereof, and for us to oppose it, or attempt to alter his dispensations, is contrary to reason, and must be offensive to God. Any other theory must be conceived in ignorance, nurtured and supported by crime, which makes a man unworthy of this earth, and unfits him for a future state.

More may be learned from the beasts of the field, and the fowls of the air, than the imagination of man would conceive. I have walked among and observed them, and from the experiments I have made in the vegetable kingdom, hath originated my limited share of knowledge. My system is not founded on theory but practice; not from the study of books, but from the study of Nature; and observations derived from the face of the earth and from the animal creation.

> "See man from Nature rising slow to art!
> To copy Instinct then was Reason's part;
> Thus then to man the voice of Nature 'spake
> Go, from the creatures thy instructions take;
> Learn from the beasts the physic of the field;
> Learn from the birds what food the thickets yield;
> The art of building from the bee receive;
> Learn of the mole to plough, the worm to weave;
> Learn of the little nautilus to sail,
> Spread the thin oar, and catch the rising gale:
> Here too all forms of social union find,
> And thus let Reason late instruct mankind."
>   DR. GOLDSMITH.

"for the smallest of the Creator's works are every way complete."

If Dioscor, Bellonius, Dioscorides, or Galen, so many years since their scientific labours, were to rise from the dead and walk into my study, and inquire of me what useful discoveries have been made in Nature's medicine since their time, I should feel somewhat ashamed, and not very well know how to reply. These once clear and deep-thinking botanists would have occasion to say: *"What you have effected in the course of so many years is not very considerable, or equal to the improvements of other arts and sciences; therefore bestir yourselves - we shall now lay ourselves down to sleep again, and trust you will not sleep away the next hundred years."*

It is really humiliating that so many years have passed away, and no safe discovery made for the *cure of Gout*. How many of the first men in the land have claimed the credit of making the first discovery, or some improvement, by the introduction of *colchicum*! Yet I think the liberal part of the profession, those who may not agree with my views on any other point, will allow that colchicum is to be dreaded for its deleterious effects, however the preparation may be, whether used as the root, the seed, or the leaf. I consider it my positive duty to warn the public against the use of colchicum, witnessing, as I have, the lamentable results of using this medicine, which acts so powerfully on the fibres and nerves as to bring on apoplexy, epilepsies, palsies, loss of memory, and the like. What are they but the worst of quacks, who introduce medicines so fatal in their consequences as this vile colchicum! Read what Sir Charles Scudamore has said on this powerful poison, (and it is probable that he has had experience of it. He says, *"Tincture of Colchicum, the preparation of Hellebore and Opium, Wilson's Tincture, and Reynolds' Specific, do in most instances for a few trials influence the local symptoms very speedily; but, so far from removing the cause of gout, they leave the disposition to the disease much stronger in the system, with less power, it is true, to produce violent inflammatory attack, and lead to the still more calamitous, because more constant sufferings of the chronic form of the disease. The patient emphatically describes that his feelings put him in constant dread of something worse occurring than the gout, which his constitution seems no longer able fairly to produce. With the effects of electerium and opium I am the least acquainted, but I have abundant opportunities to know that each of the other medicines sooner or later disappoint the patient of his expected ease, rendering merely a palliative assistance, and keeping the disease dormant for a time only, so that it is left to prey on the constitution with more lasting and serious ill effects."*

Is it not criminal, I would ask, to use this dreadful poison, when there are so many substitutes (as I can and have offered to prove) to be found among our most common plants? One of the many I use is daily eaten from the plate of almost every family in France; it is perfectly safe, and requires only forty hours to do that which colchicum certainly does in five, but always with danger. My remedy, as my patients can prove, while it cures, strengthens the solids, and produces a vigorous vibration and circulation of the blood, causing a good digestion, by a separation and carrying off the grosser humours, thereby preventing an early relapse. All kinds of rheumatic pains brought under my observation and treatment have given way, under the powerful agency of my medicated vapour baths, properly impregnated with such herbs as will remove the cause of disease from the most remote parts. It is the duty of every practitioner to avoid giving anything to force nature - assist her he may; and even in this: much caution should be used, and as soon as the intention is answered he must cease.

I have not at any time depended on the opinions of others: the volume of nature I found best suited to my taste. The field lay open before me; in my rambles I struck into a new path of enquiry, and have broken new ground, both in the cultivation and practice of English medicine, and intend some day, if my life is spared, to endeavour to show the world that almost every plant on the face of the earth carries the mark or seal for the disorders which it cures.

Let us bear in mind that the saying of holy writ, *"by their fruits ye shall know them,"* is at least applicable to plants as to the human species. The brute creation knows by instinct what is good and what is hurtful to them, for nature is pure as it came from its divine author: it delights in simplicity, and is the teacher of only such valuable truths as serve to promote it. Nature, like truth, is simple and uniform: to follow Nature is an excellent and a safe rule. I was much pleased on reading the sound advice which Baron Portal gave to his brother physicians: he says, "Nature is admirable in the means which she makes use of for the preservation of the beings whom she has created, especially in *cases of diseases.* She ought to be minutely considered, in order to follow her operations, and to second them; and woe to the physician (he might have added, patient!) who does not take her for the guide of his conduct."

It is a melancholy fact, that in the present day diseases are more numerous and inveterate than ever existed before. Many in the profession are a set of idle and shallow men, wishing to make a short cut into physic, without the trouble of studying Nature's medicine, as did their forefathers. They despise pharmacy and botany, cry down hypothesis, and confound distempers. The practitioner is often so mercenary as to make his profession a *mere trade*; be runs to his patient in haste, asks a few general questions, scribbles out one of his hacknied prescriptions, takes his fee, and away to the next, whom he treats in the same way. He should certainly allow sufficient time and thought to find out the nature and cause of his patient's distemper, and superintend personally the preparation of his own prescriptions. Few persons are aware of the consequences of the present system of trusting the mixture of these medicines to inexperienced apprentices and others: at present we purchase medicines as we would brimstone to make matches.

> "O, place and greatness, millions of false eyes
> Are stuck upon thee: volumes of report
> Run with these false and most contrarious quest
> Upon thy doings! Thousand sallies of wit
> Make thee the father of their idle dream,
> And rack thee in their fancies."   SHAKSPEARE

EXAMPLES OF NATURAL GENIUS.

"Pray, now, no more. My mother,
Who has a privilege to extol her blood,
When she does praise me grieves me. I have done
As you have done, that's what I can, induced,
As you have been, that's for my country.
Heaven doth with us as we with torches do;
Not light them for themselves - for if our virtues
Did not go forth of us, ' twere all alike
As if we had them not. Spirits are not finely touched
But for high purposes; nor Nature never lends
The smallest scruple of her excellence;
But, like a thrifty goddess, she determines
Herself the glory of a creditor
Both of thanks and interest."
                                    SHAKSPEARE.

THERE may be, even in this enlightened age, an illiterate few, reluctant to admit that the mind of man may, by a particular endowment of Nature, be so stored with the rudiments of science, as to arrive at once to that stage of excellence, which another must reach by dint of severe and long-continued study. Did Shakspeare excel in dramatic poetry, only in the ratio in which his education excelled that of all other writers? Is not the reverse the fact?

A catalogue might be made of the shifts many others have had before me to enjoy their darling study. Ferguson was put to a trade which Nature had not intended him for; but his talent discovered to him the situation of the stars by means of a thread with a few beads strung on it; and Tycho Brahé did the same with a pair of compasses.

The self-taught Rittenhouse, when employed as a farm-labourer, used to draw geometrical diagrams on his plough, and study them as he turned up the furrow. Pascal, when a mere boy, made himself master of the elementary propositions of geometry without the aid of a master, by tracing figures on the floor of his room with a bit of coal. This, or a stick burned at the end, has often been the young painter's first pencil.

Mr. John Davy, when only six years old, began to imitate the church bells with eight horse-shoes suspended from the ceiling with strings in such a manner as to form an octave. Sir Humphrey Davy first published his chemical studies without teacher or guide, aided only by the scantiest and rudest apparatus. The father of the celebrated Barry sent him to sea because he disapproved of the son's favourite study; even that would not do, as his greatest pleasure was to cover the deck with sketches of objects made with chalk or ochre. He once exclaimed to a companion: *"I could be happy, on going home, to find some corner where I could sit down in the midst of my studies, where I might have models of nature, when necessary, bread and soup, and a coat to cover me."* Bloomfield is another instance of self-tuition, as he could scarce read or write on his arrival in London. The late Benjamin West first showed his talent while watching a child that lay asleep in its cradle, when with paper, pen and ink only, he made a drawing of the face. When his mother and sister returned and saw it, the former exclaimed, *"I declare he has made a likeness of Little Sally! "* The first brush be ever used was made from the hairs of a cat's tail, having no other. That celebrated surgeon, Hunter, worked as a carpenter until he was twenty seven years of age. Mr. Samuel Parks, the well-known author of the Chemical Catechism, the Rudiments of Chemistry, &c. was a grocer at Stoke-upon-Trent until he was forty-two years of age; but the fruit of his private labours, which the grocery business could not despoil him of, he at last turned to an excellent account. I could name many men of the first talent who had not been taught to read or write: this shows the powerful work of Providence, by forming men in different moulds, and placing them afterwards in different circumstances, so that philosophy and art shall not be left uncultivated, but that there should be labourers to engage in each pursuit.

> "So work the honey bees;
> Creatures that, by a rule in nature, teach
> The act of order to a peopled kingdom.
> They have a king, and officers of different degrees,
> Where some, like magistrates, correct at home;
> Others, like merchants, venture trade abroad,
> Others, like soldiers, armed in their stings,
> Make boot upon the summer's velvet buds,
> Which pillage they with merry march bring home
> To the tent royal of their emperor;
> Who, busied in his majesty, surveys
> The singing masons building roofs of gold;
> The sober grave citizens kneading up the honey;
> The poor mechanic porters crowding in
> Their heavy burdens at his narrow gate;
> The sad-eye justice, with his surly hum,
> Delivering over to executioners pale
> The lazy yawning drone."
>   SHAKSPEARE.

Let lordly man take a lesson from the economy of a bee-hive! Every man has the power to educate himself in that station of life for which nature intends him; and that this power is not confined to any particular acquirement. How necessary is it that this truth should be diffused and felt through out all classes of society: how would it encourage the children of poverty and neglect to use every effort to educate themselves. Would not this feeling help to smooth the roughest of their difficulties, and to give them new strength to emancipate themselves from the ignorance in which they were reared? Such as are

> "Well compound with gifts of Nature, flowing and swelling over with arts and exercise."
>   SHAKSPEARE.

Many have failed who, had they had this assurance, might have led to attainments beneficial to themselves and mankind! I again say, this feeling would soon lead the young mind from unprofitable and corruptive pleasures, to that of a *natural* relish for *intellectual* enjoyments - such as I have enjoyed even during a stolen half-hour from business. Time and talents are gifts that every man will have to account for. Talent may not be given to all alike, but time is; the day is the same length for each of us, and by no contrivance can we lengthen or shorten it one moment; we must spend it either for something or nothing. We often see the young and rich man, who can live without any exertion on his part, lose the power of exerting himself to that degree which is necessary for the acquisition of knowledge; for his money provides him with vain and useless enjoyments: every man must see by the present march of intellect that the great power which Nature has given to man has never yet been put to the stretch; we are all capable of much more than we are aware of.

It would be folly in myself to lay claim to more than the ability born with me, and an active reflecting mind. A humble village education is all I can pretend to; and so perhaps might Shakspeare himself have said. It is, at all events, singular that, with the limited education I received, I should have become a passionate admirer of Shakspeare. It was by mere accident his works were put into my hand. I was so charmed with them, that my young and active mind eagerly imbibed the principles they contained for every age and condition of life. I read them so often, that before I was fifteen I was familiar with the largest portion of his works. In fact, for years Shakspeare's writings were my only companion; therefore, without any presumption on my part, I may lay claim to him for my schoolmaster and instructor in the affairs of life. It was he who told me, when describing money:

> "All that glistens is not gold,
> Often have you heard that told;
> Many a man his life hath sold
> But for my outside to behold."

Again he says:

> "Thus much of this, will make black, white; foul, fair;
> Wrong, right; base, noble; old, young; coward, valiant;
> Will lug your priests and servants from your sides.
> This yellow slave
> Will knit and break religions; bless the accurs'd;
> Make the hoar leprosy ador'd; place thieves,
> And give them title, knee, and approbation,
> With senators on the bench."

It was he who taught me to believe that *"there is a tide in the affairs of men, which taken at the flood leads on to fortune:"* from his writings I learnt that *"to wilful men the injuries that they themselves procure must be their schoolmasters:"* it was he that in formed me that *"he cannot be a perfect man not being tried and tutored in the world:"* and *"experience is by industry achieved, and perfected by the swift course of time."* He taught me to believe that there *"is a divinity that shapes our ends, rough-hew them how we will;"* and made me feel that *"mine honour keeps the weather of my fate."* It was he who said that *"ignorance is the characteristic of childhood, and the mind that is uninformed, at whatever period of life, is still in an infant state;"* and that *"the love of human kind will make you a friend to every human creature."* Shakspeare declares the grand truth, that *"the life of a man has many cares belonging to it; but the first and greatest care is that of the immortal soul, and to place any other in the scale against it would be absolute folly."* He tells us, that in the world *"there lurks a still and dumb discoursive devil, that tempts most cunningly - but be not tempted."* It was Shakspeare who taught me to say, *"I am a true labourer: I earn what I eat, get what I wear, owe no man hate, envy no man's happiness, glad of other men's good;"* and that *"one man in his time plays many a part;"* and that *"when we enter upon the stage of life we must be prepared for the changes of the scene."* And does he not put us on our guard, by telling us that *"some men think others honest that only seem to be so."* Yes, this man has shown us so much of human nature, that it must be in her school he studied; and to his honour we find that every thing which is good and great, or even worth our seeking for, is arrayed on the side of religion and morality. It may appear strange that, being so great an admirer of Shakspeare, I never saw one of his plays performed until I was twenty-three years old, and never but one from that time to the present.

I may, perhaps, be excused stating, in a very few words, in what way I obtained the most important portion of what anatomical knowledge I possess, the more especially as it will shew the means by which Providence sometimes ordains, that some events which at the first view appear to us unmitigated calamities, may ultimately tend to our material benefit. When young, I met with so severe an accident, that recovery was considered nearly hopeless. I was placed under the care of a most eminent surgeon, and recovered; but residing for eighteen months under his roof, and having constant access to his museum and library, I acquired the groundwork of that anatomical knowledge which, strengthened from other sources, has since been of such essential service to me.

Nature, it is well known, is extremely capricious in the bestowal of some of her choicest gifts, and no doubt, had I relied altogether on acquired knowledge, my success might have been more limited. We have often seen persons of humble origin, guided by the dictates of nature and reason, arriving at exceeding clever discoveries, so benevolent is the Almighty to his creatures in every station of life. Parents would do well to study the natural inclinations of their children in their tender years. Is it not reasonable to suppose that it arises from some natural congeniality between the heart and mind? As plants prefer certain climates, may we not conclude that there is some connexion be tween the climate and plant? So it is between the moral and intellectual endowments of mankind. We shall find, if we examine the characters of those persons who, from the exertion of their own talents, have raised themselves from comparative obscurity to opulence, that this must be the case.

My foible has always been close study, to find out by what means the productions of the earth are suitable to the wants of human life, both for food and medicine: *"Behold I have given you every herb bearing seed, and every tree bearing fruit, and to you it shall be for meat;"* and I now cannot but come to this conclusion, that the practice of medicine is bad, and one hundred years behind every other art and science; and there are very few medical men but will acknowledge this. To many of them I beg leave to return my most grateful thanks for the kindness I have received from them, both in their personal friendships, and the liberality of mind they have shown in transferring to me patients whom they knew I could speedily relieve. This reciprocity of good feeling has been of mutual interest, as I have frequently sent patients to medical men of this metropolis, when applied to for my advice in diseases which I do not profess to understand, and such cases have frequently occurred. I will give one recent case, to show that I never tamper with a disease that I do not understand, or while there is the hope of honourable men in the profession doing good. A gentleman of title and high rank in the army arrived at my house in October last from his country seat; on examining him, I found that instead of gout in the stomach, it was inflammation of the lungs. I sent for a medical gentleman to attend him at my house; also that worthy man, Dr. Nevinson, who is an honour to his profession, was called in, and with their united assistance, in one week he was enabled to return to his town residence, where I have had the honour of paying him almost daily friendly visits. While I write this I have two gentlemen from Cambridge in my house as patients; one of their cases is entirely out of my practice, nor should I have undertaken it but that the first medical men in Cambridge had reported him incurable. (In all these difficult cases I invite medical men to my house, to witness my mode of cure, and some days I receive many visits from them, for this purpose. They confess the treatment is quite unknown to them, yet still they approve of it, and I trust with many of them, that the time is not far distant when it will be in general practice.) This patient leaves me in a few days: to use his own words, he *"would astonish the doctors when he got home."* They would be more astonished if they knew by what simple means the cure was effected, with the assistance only of sixteen medicated baths. I showed this case to a medical gentleman on the first day, who gave me little hopes; but when I told him I should endeavour to attain a certain effect, and the herbs I should use for that purpose, *"Oh!"* said he, *"if you succeed in accomplishing that object you may effect a cure, but not else."* The Countess of (Blank) sent one of her servants to me who had been helpless nine years. I did not hold out a probability of success, unless I could accomplish a certain point; this was done so quickly, that her Ladyship sent her medical adviser to see him at my house. At the end of twelve days his surprise was great at seeing the man walk about the room. I mentioned what means I had used, and what herbs I had put into the bath. He then said: *"Mr. Tilke, the more I see and hear, the more I am astonished; and my opinion is, that you have such judgment in the use of herbs, that you can accomplish whatever you undertake."* (Mr. Russell, builder, of Blackheath, has wished me to say he was present at this interview.) The medical gentleman repeated to her Ladyship nearly the same words, as she called on me the same day, to say how delighted he was with his interview, and that he would call on me again. Let any practitioner shew him self equal to such extremely difficult cases, he will have no occasion to hold out baits for patients by advertisements; which, in fact, I have never done, as I have not altered my original opinion, namely, that if my treatment was good, it would find its own level. My patients come to me recommended by others, to whom I have given relief. I keep a journal of all cases, and of the means adopted for their cure, with the omission of names only for the sake of delicacy; which amount at present to more than five hundred in the neighbourhood of London; and should it not be published during my life-time, I shall make arrangements that it shall at some time appear, for the good of society at large. When this is done, medical as well as non-medical men will be astonished to find all has been accomplished by simple English herbs. In every case I give the manner of preparing them. Dr. John Gregory, in an essay on the office and duties of a physician, remarks that *"the affectation of concealing the medical art retarded its progress, rendered it suspicious, and tended to draw ridicule and disgrace upon its professors."* Many will blame me for making the public (as they say) too wise :

"But alas! it is my vice, my fault, while others fish with craft for great opinion, and with equal truth catch mere simplicity: while some with cunning gild their copper crowns, with truth and plainness I do wear mine." - SHAKSPEARE

SHORT ACCOUNT

OF THE

PROPERTIES OF HERBS AND ROOTS.

DANDELION. (*Heptodon*). - This plant grows in abundance in all parts of Europe; taken any way it is a good aperient as well as diuretic; the young leaves are very good in salads, or eaten with bread and butter; and knowing well the properties of this herb, I am compelled to make the same remark as I have done elsewhere in this book, that Nature has given those things most bountifully which are most useful; this plant is an instance, as it is in perfection all the year round, and there is no disease but what it will soothe; by its drying and temperate qualities, one ounce of the expressed juice a day, by perseverance, will cure the dropsy; it eases pain, and procures rest and sleep to bodies that are distracted. It is highly spoken of by French physicians, who are more alive to the properties of vegetable medicine, and more liberal in communicating knowledge, than the English are.

ROSEMARY. (*Rosmarinus.*) - Both flowers and leaves of this plant will strengthen the brain, and help dim eyes; made into oils or ointments, it will recover cold or benumbed joints and sinews; it comforts the heart, and raiseth the spirits.

RUE. (*Ruta.*) - This plant, when in perfection, which is in June, is good to cause and quicken the circulation of the blood, and to dissolve gross humours; four ounces of the leaves may be taken at bed-time as an infusion, which will be found a sure remedy for that troublesome visitor the nightmare; an ointment made with oil of roses and vinegar cureth St. Anthony's fire, and all running ulcers. Can any botanist tell the reason why this root and sweet basil will not grow near each other?

SAGE. (*Salvia*). This excellent herb, taken any way, and for any disease, must do good, and for this reason, it strengthens the head, nerves, cures trembling of the limbs, and promotes a strong circulation of the fluids. The Chinese wonder we should buy their tea, when we have so much sage and speedwell of our own growth, which they consider by far the best. The public ought to be made acquainted with the fact, that a great quantity of those two herbs are exported for the use of those shrewd people; who laugh, (and well enough they may,) at the exchange for the wretched stuff they send us, which they have so properly named slow poison.

SCURVY-GRASS. (*Cochlearia*).- Scurvy under various forms is common in this country, and this grass is such a sovereign remedy against it that it cannot be too highly spoken of. In April or May, when this herb is in season, it might be mixed with sorrel, or any other acid herb, and eaten as a salad. When scurvy- grass cannot be got, water-dock or spearpint-dock may be used in its stead, made into an infusion,

MANDRAKE. (*Atropa*). - This is a most useful, but neglected herb; the roots boiled with ivy and oil heal St. Anthony's fire; the green leaves bruised with lard and barley meal heal all hot swellings and imposthumes an infusion given as a lavement, easeth the piles and causeth sleep. Shakspeare seems to have been aware of its being soporific, as he makes Iago exclaim, after arousing the jealousy of Othello:

> "Not poppy, nor mandragora, (mandrake)
> Nor all the drowsy syrups of the world,
> Shall ever medicine thee to that sweet sleep
> Which thou hadst yesterday."

By this it appears it was formerly given by our forefathers as a syrup, to ease pain and cause sleep. I have given it in doses of three, four, or five grains in powder of the root for the same purpose; I have also placed a piece of the root on the pillow of my patients, as the smell only causes sound sleep. This only relates to the male: the properties of the female are very different. If this cause too much stupor, dip a sponge in vinegar, and hold it to the nose.

SHEPHERD'S PURSE. (*Thlaspi*). - This is another proof that Providence has made the most useful plant the most common, and Nature in her bounty has allowed them to flower all the summer, and they sometimes flower twice a year; common sense therefore would point it out for general use; instead of which, it seems man neglects them. Few plants possess more virtue than this, which I am sorry to say, up to this time, is utterly disregarded. An infusion of this herb is a gentle and safe astringent, good in all fevers, inferior to nothing for the piles, or a habitual purging; a wine-glass full of the juice of the leaves, with one of red wine, will check and soothe the overflowings of any kind in man or woman. In my rides in the lanes round London, how often have I been grieved to see this excellent and useful herb thrown over the hedge, and trampled under foot, as if it were perfectly useless. Shepherd's purse, tormentil, and comfrey, are near alike; I only wish those three herbs, together or separate, were fairly tried for the cholera; it is not yet too late. Let the profession look back to the ancients, who saw the good effects of those medicines, and have shown us the doses and manner of giving them. I have found them always right, and they may be depended upon for our best guides. Like every other art, much may be learned from a careful trial. Mothers, consider this and the next herb for the use of your daughters, and esteem it as a valuable secret. If this hint conveys to my readers the advantage of such simple medicine, I shall consider my time in stating it has been well employed.

MUGWORT. (*Arlemisia.*) - The leaves and flowers are all full of virtue; they are aromatic to the taste, and a most safe and excellent medicine in all female disorders, and Providence has placed it in every part of the land. There is no medicine to equal this for safety and certainty for young women, or in fact at any time of life, when the efforts of nature are too weak. Nothing can be more destructive to the constitution than the use of powerful drugs; for *"it is not proper to weaken her who is already too weak."* On this occasion pick the flowers and buds from the tops of the stalks, and take one ounce, and the same of *carduus benedictus,* or holy-thistle, all cut small, and put into a jug; put one pint of boiling water upon it; when cool it is to be drank with a little honey; this may be taken every day. Should any further help be required, a few days before the indisposition is expected, put one pound of mugwort and half an ounce of socotrine aloes, boil it in two gallons of water for twenty minutes; put all in a pan, and sit over it as warm as possible every night until all is well; if mugwort cannot be got, tansy or feverfew will do nearly as well.

LIQUORICE. (*Glycyrrhiza*). - This is a fine medicine, and deserves more praise than I can bestow upon it. An infusion of the fresh roots is excellent to take off the acrimony of the humours. In coughs alone it is, as a remedy, without its equal; it promotes expectoration, and at the same time thickens the juices. Excellent for dropsy, as it abates thirst. This is singular, as every other sweet increases it; the sweet of liquorice is equal to that of sugar; the former checks thirst, the latter increases it; a trial will show this to be perfectly true. Many plants of less virtue are more celebrated, but there are few deserve a fairer trial.

FIG-TREE. (*Ficus*). – The juice from the green leaves, melted with lard, equal parts, will make an excellent ointment for deafness, put into the ear on a little cotton. I hardly know a better remedy for the leprosy than than this. It also clears the face of scurf and pimples, it heals all fretting ulcers, and is good for inflamed eyes.

TORMENTIL. (*Tormentilla*). - It is deserving the name of English sarsaparilla. I think I cannot do better than repeat what Dr. Thornton has said of it, as I have proved the same to be fact. He says: *"I have witnessed extraordinary cures performed by this root. I knew a poor man fond of botanical excursions, who either by tradition or accident knew the powers of this root, and by making a strong decoction sweetened with honey, he cured agues, which had resisted Peruvian bark, long standing diarrhœas, ulcers of the legs, turned out of hospitals incurable; the worst scorbutic ulcers, and confluent smallpox; the hooping-cough, fluxes. This poor man had so much practice as to excite the attention of Lord William Russell, who allowed him a piece of ground in his park to cultivate the plant, which he kept as a secret."* So much says Dr. Thornton. Now I have found half an ounce of this root, two drachms of hops, and one pint of water, taken every day, do wonders for the piles and bowel complaint. The powder of the root mixed with vinegar, and spread on oil silk, and laid on the loins, will assist those who cannot from weakness hold their water; the same will dissolve all kernels about the ears, throat, and jaws; also the king's evil, as it is called, by restraining the sharp humours that flow to them.

BORAGE, (*Borago*) - Fumitory, (*Fumaria*) - and ELDER (*Sambucus*). - The properties of these three are so nearly alike in fevers, that to save space I shall describe them under one head; and indeed, if I had the ability as I have the will, and the knowledge of these safe medicines, I could write a book larger than this on their virtues, and if these, as well as many other useful plants, could only be imported from some distant parts, and sold at extravagant prices, there is no doubt that they would be held in great estimation. The productions of Nature are given to man for food and medicine; common, cheap, and easy to be found, but the medicine of the doctors of the present day are dear, and scarce to be found, and hardly worth the finding. These three herbs are all great cordials, and strengtheners of nature, excellent to defend the heart, and to resist and expel the poisons or venom of putrid and pestilential fever; they will expel melancholy, clarify the blood, and mitigate heat in fever; together they will cure the yellow jaundice and dropsy, which they expel by urine in great abundance; they expel phlegm and choler, and those saltish, choleric, and malignant humours, which cause leprosy, scabs, tetters, and such-like breakings-out of the skin. After having performed these and many other services, they strengthen all the inward parts of man, and leave none of the wreck of the disease behind, as we too often see in fevers, according to the practice of the school of medicine. Let them no longer be allowed then to rot in the earth, if you love your fellow-creature, if you love your children, if you love your health, and if you love your ease, and if you can afford it, always keep them in a syrup, or by you in any way; when you see or know a case of fever, give it to your afflicted neighbour as freely as I bestow my studies on them; and if you do not find them relieved blame me and no other.

WOOD BETONY. (*Betonica*). Ought to be gathered in May. This herb boiled with wine or water is good for those who cannot digest their meals; or have belchings and a continual rising in their stomach. A drachm of the root in powder, mixed with honey and vinegar, taken every day, is good for those who have a rupture in their urinary glands, and pass blood with their water. The green herb bruised with lard makes an excellent ointment for wounds, old sores, or ulcers; for the latter add a little salt and figs bruised together; it a good and useful herb, and very proper to be kept in every man's house, either dry, in syrup, conserve, or in ointment.

BUCKTHORN (*Rhumnus*). The properties of this are exceedingly like the wood betony.

PELLITORY OF THE WALL (*Parietaria.*) — If this is planted in a shady place it will afterwards spring up of its own accord, time June and July; the seed is ripe soon after. A decoction of this herb, with honey, is excellent for an old dry cough, shortness of breath, or wheezing in the throat. About three ounces of the juice, (or which is more easy to make a strong decoction,) taken at a time, helps the stoppage of urine, and expels stone or gravel in the kidneys or bladder, which cause pains in the loins, sides, or bowels; the juice bruised with a little salt is effectual to cleanse fistulas or green wounds, and to heal them up safely; the juice made into a syrup, with honey, and a desert-spoonful taken every morning fasting, is very good for the dropsy. Feed a goat entirely on this, or any other herb that it will eat and is fond of, and drink plenty of the milk, it will answer every purpose. The root, burnt to a powder, is good to whiten teeth; the juice, held in the mouth, eases pain of the gums proceeding from rheumatism.

WILD TANSY, OR SILVER WEED (*Potentilla*). -The time June and July; a decoction, with honey, will expel wind in the stomach and bowels; if often smelled to it will relieve the head-ache; if boiled in olive oil and well rubbed in, it is good for the sinews shrunk by cramps, pains, weakness, and stiffness of the joints, after repeated attacks of the gout. The same, mixed with a little bee's-wax , is an excellent salve for wounds.

GROUND IVY (*Glechoma*).- The best time is May, but unless the winter be very sharp it may be gathered all the year round; it is quick, sharp, and bitter in taste. An excellent medicine for all inward wounds, ulcerated lungs, or other parts; the decoction may be improved by boiling equal parts of rosemary, mixed with honey; it will ease griping pains, and windy choleric humours in the stomach; it will cure the yellow jaundice by opening the pores of the gall and liver; it gives ease to those who are troubled with the sciatica, or the gout in the hands, knees, or feet; this herb has the same effect with beast as with man.

SARSAPARILLA (*Smilax*). - This is a foreign plant. The true herb is considered not to heat, but rather to dry the humours, and waste them away by a secret and hidden property which it contains; with perseverance it will ease, and often cure, all pains of the sinews or joints, all running sores in the legs, all tumours, swellings, spots, and fullness of the skin, by purifying the blood. An excellent diet drink may be made in the following manner: take gum guaicum one ounce, bark of the same one ounce, sassafras one ounce, sarsaparilla two ounces, juniper berries half an ounce, simmer all in two quarts of water for two hours, then strain and add one drachm of cinnamon, and make it to please the palate with liquorice or honey. This quantity is sufficient for two days.

SPEEDWELL (*Veronica*). - If this herb was to be sent by the Chinese for green tea we should hardly know to the contrary. This herb is very like the wood betony; together they make an excellent beverage for breakfast.

BALM (*Melissa.*) - Time, June, July, and August. The juice is good for green wounds, melted in a small quantity of lard. Serapio says, *"a strong effusion, often drank, causeth the mind to be merry, and reviveth the heart when faint. Good for those who have weak digestions!"* Pounded with suet it is good to remove wens, keruels, or hard swellings in the flesh or throat; the herb, when green, bruised with a little linseed oil and laid warm on a boil, will ripen and break it; it is also good to sweeten the breath if made and drank as tea, with a little cream of tartar or lemon juice.

CHAMOMILE. (*Anthemis.*) - The wild flowers that grow on the heath of this well-known plant are the most valuable; made into tea, and a cupfull taken in the morning fasting, is good to fortify the stomach, and create an appetite, and prevents the wind and heartburn. They are excellent for fomentations, as they will disperse congealed blood in bruises, tumours, and swellings.

PELLITORY OF SPAIN (*Pyrethrum*). - This is a foreign plant. One ounce of the juice, taken in a wine-glass full of Hollands, one hour before a fit of the ague comes on, will cure it after three or four doses; the herb, or the root chewed in the mouth, purgeth the brain of phlegmatic humours. The powder of the root, snuffed up the nostrils, eases the head-ache, by distilling the humour of the brain. But above all it will cure the tooth-ache, which knowledge, to sufferers with this pain, is worth twenty times the price of this little book. Take one ounce of the root, cut it small, put it to half a pint of gin in a bottle, let it stand in a warm place; shake it repeatedly for two or three days, then strain it, and when there is pain in the teeth or gums put a teaspoonful of the mixture on the part affected, and keep it there as long as possible. This rubbed on the head will cure the pain thereof, but the herb, or the root chewed in the mouth, will do nearly as well.

CINQUEFOIL, or five-finger grass (*potentilla*). -Time, June and May. This is so much like tormentil that I have but few remarks to make. An infusion is excellent for the liver, comforts the stomach, and will cure the jaundice; the root boiled in vinegar will heal the shingles, sores of all kinds, and cancerous ulcers.

MEDLARS (*Mespilus*). Time for the flowers in May. The fruit is ripe in September and October. The fruit is good to stay all fluxes of blood in man or woman; very proper to be eaten by the latter when in a state of pregnancy, as it will prevent and cure their longings after unnatural meats, &c. The medlar stones, made into a powder and drank in wine, will break and expel the stones, and is a perfect cure for the gravel, if only persevered in.

ST. JOHN'S WORT (H*ypericum*).- Time, July and August. I have found this herb, as well as many others I use, have a wonderful effect on patients in my steam-bath, who have been in the habit of taking mercury; on their inhaling the vapour it seems to set all the humours in a state of fermentation, even to bringing on a slight degree of salivation. Two drachms of the seed of this herb, pounded and put into broth, will expel congealed blood from the stomach, occasioned by the bursting of a vein, bruises, falls, &c.; also easeth pains of the loins. In America they are blessed with this herb growing among their corn, which makes it much superior to the English. From the excellent properties I know it to contain, I believe that, ground with the wheat, and eaten as bread, it would prove a cure, or preventative, against many of the diseases man is heir to. This flour, it is well known by almost every baker who works in his business, improves the quality of the bread by having a small quantity of it in every batch, particularly in seasons when the English flour is of inferior quality. This flour, as we are informed by a very clever author, contains *one-fourth* more gluton than our famous wheats grown in Gloucestershire, known by the name of *rivets;* the only objection I ever heard, during the years I attended Mark-lane, was from its *smell,* which the trade called *savey,* I consider it more like *rosin.* The juice of this herb is of a reddish kind, which gives that beautiful yellow bloom to the flour so much admired by the trade: to whom I will make a few plain remarks publicly, such as I have privately made to many of my friends, *viz.* when they use this flour, or any other that is rich and glutinous, they should give the dough more proof than for common English flour, because from the great quantity of *glutinous* matter it contains, if it is not well fermented, it will not spring or rise in the oven, nor will it be so digestible to the stomach, for in the process of fermentation the saccharine matter becomes sufficiently divided, and then the heat of the oven throws off the superfluous quantity of acid it contains, thus preventing the bread causing a fermentation in the stomach of those who eat it, as this will constipate the bowels, inflame the blood, and produce fever. Few men living have had greater opportunities, or perhaps have given their time more to fermentation than I have, always considering it a most important part of my business: which I believe to be the reason I gained so much credit in the execution of many contracts I have had with Government for the supply of bread, the prime article of life. Every experiment I make, and they are not a few, convinces me that the knowledge of fermentation is yet in its infancy.

HOLY THISTLE.

"Get you some of this distilled *carduus benedictus*, and lay it to your heart; it is the only thing for a qualm. I mean plain holy thistle."

SHAKSPEARE.

From the above it appears the immortal bard knew the wonderful properties of this herb. Some botanists have called it *Blessed Thistle*; those names were given to it, no doubt, on account of its excellent qualities. As I do so much with this herb in private practice, I at first did not feel, in justice to myself, that I ought, at present, to publish the virtues with which God has indeed blessed it. But when my heart intends a kindness, I do not like, as Lord Hastings says, "To let the coldness of delay hang on it." I can state as a fact, that I have caused more of this herb to be used in the last four years than was consumed in London in fifty years previously. I shall have very little to say of it myself, as I intend to give the opinions of others two or three hundred years since; and I can assure my readers, although the robust health of man has degenerated from that time, the properties of this excellent herb have not; I have found it such a clarifier of the blood, that by drinking an infusion once or twice a-day, sweetened with honey, instead of tea, it would be a perfect cure for the headache, or what is sometimes called the meagrims; in fact, this plant has very great power in the purification and circulation of the blood, from the bad state of which arise all the humours of the body: and although, in another page, I have expressed the opinion that we are different from each other, in every sense of the word, only in proportion as these humours abound more or less in each of us, yet, retaining this opinion, I do believe this herb must benefit every constitution.

"The why is as plain as the way to the parish church."

SHAKSPEARE.

By the great effect it has on the blood, it comforts the *pia mater* of the brain, by which it must strengthen the sense and memory; it will also cleanse and mollify an infected stomach, which must produce good blood, and good blood cannot but produce good and healthy secretions: it is also good for the dropsy or ague, neither of which can exist if the circulation of the blood be pure. I should advise every mother to give this to her daughter from the age of ten to twenty: my reason I need not give, only that it may prevent them from years of pain and misery. I will now give what Mattheolus and Fuschius have written of carduus benedictus. *"It is,"* they say, *"a plant of great virtue; it helpeth inwardly and outwardly; it strengthens all the principal members of the body, as the brain, the heart, the stomach, the liver, the lungs, and the kidneys; it is also a preservative against all disease, for it causes perspiration, by which the body is purged of much corruption. Such as breedeth diseases it expelleth the venom of infection; it consumes and wasteth away all bad humours, therefore give God thanks for his goodness, who hath given this herb and all others for the benefit of our health."* Holy thistle may be used in four ways: first, it may be eaten in the green leaf with bread and butter for breakfast (instead of water cresses); 2dly, The leaves may be dried and made into a powder, and a drachm taken in wine or otherwise every day; 3dly, A wine glass of the juice may be taken every day; 4thly, (which is the way I should recommend,) is in infusion about two ounces of the dried plant simmered in a quart of water for two hours. This medicine given in this way the daintiest stomach will not refuse; if the seeds of this plant are sown again in September or October, clear of a north-east wind, you may have the herb green summer and winter. Those who have gardens I would advise to attend to this; any soil will produce it in abundance; it may be taken any time as a preventative; but to remove disease, used going to bed is best, as it will, after a few times taken, most likely cause a copious perspiration. I shall do my best, when time will allow, to bring this plant into so general a use, that I hope to see it grown common in our fields, then I shall feel that I have discovered and communicated the only grand secret worth knowing in this life: *viz* . how one man may contrive to be more useful in life than another - all the rest is mere moonshine. Time for gathering flowers for preserving is July or August; but you may gather the young buds early in the spring (March, April, and May), and use it almost any way, and it will change your blood as the season changes, which common sense tells us is a very sure way to preserve health. Any of the other thistles may be used as substitutes, such as the common thistle, fullers thistle, melancholy thistle, our lady's thistle, woolly or cotton thistle; they are all purifiers of the blood, as well as all kinds of docks; but the red-water dock is the head of the dock family, as the carduus is of the thistle family. I consider it a high privilege to be on intimate terms with both those families.

I have now given a description of a sufficient number of simple and useful herbs for almost every disease, omitting only such as would be unsafe to trust in the hands of those who have not made medicine a study. I have not ascribed more virtues to those plants than others have done before me; and which I have proved to be true by long experience. I would beg to observe, that the proper dose of all that I have here set down, is about half an ounce of the root or a quarter of an ounce of the dried herb to a pint of water, to be taken daily, unless otherwise ordered, as will be seen; but when the herb or root is green, use treble the weight. I would recommend those who wish to have cheap and safe remedies by them, to gather every plant while in the bloom, and prepare them in conserve juice, extract or syrup.

Manner of preparing the above.

I shall now give a few easy modes of preparing the above, which I have found answer very well: all other herbs spoken of in this work may be prepared in a similar way.

JUICE OF MUGWORT. - Take the fresh herb any quantity, bruise it in a stone mortar, extract the juice, and clarify it by slightly boiling it; strain again, and preserve it. Dose, one ounce three times a-day.

SYRUP OF MUGWORT. - Three pounds of the juice of mugwort clarified by boiling and straining, to three pounds of white sugar. Boil slowly to the consistence of a syrup. Dose half an ounce twice a day,

INFUSION OF GROUND IVY. - Leaves of ground ivy and colt's-foot, each one ounce; root of liquorice half an ounce, water one quart; this to be taken in one day.

SYRUP OF GROUND IVY. - Fresh leaves of ground ivy half a pound, boiling water three pounds, infuse for ten hours, then strain and add to the liquor white sugar twice its weight; boil to a syrup. Dose two ounces a- day.

To make BLACKBERRY JAM. - Take ten pounds of blackberries and five pounds of moist *foot* sugar. Bruise it together, and then boil it for one hour, keep stirring all the time; pot it; when cold pour a little of good salad oil on the top, which will keep it good for years: this way there is no waste, very little trouble, very cheap, and, what is far above all other considerations, very wholesome for either adults or children to eat on bread instead of butter, at about one-fifth of the cost.

Uses of the same.

For the following diseases I have administered the annexed simples.

Ague. - Agrimony, betony, mustard, St. John's-wort, wormwood, tormentil and marigolds.

Asthma. - Coltsfoot, horehound, mallows, sage, speedwell, little centaury, and wood betony.

For a cancerous Swelling. - A poultice of one, or all if they can be had: Comfrey, turnips, carrots, and goose- grass. Drink tormentil tea.

Cough. - Horehound, pennyroyal, tormentil, vervain, liquorice, comfrey, mullein, stramonium, and elecampane.

Consumption. — Coltsfoot, pimpernell, chickweed, speedwell, mallows, and tormentil-root.

Convulsions. - Mother-wort, valerian, piony dwarf.
Dropsy. - Wood-betony, agrimony, chervil, garlic, borage, fumitory, parsley, tansey, wormwood, crowfoot, speedwell, toad-flax, dandelion, and pellitory wall.

To help Digestion. - Horseradish, lovage, hyssop, sage, wood-betony, buckthorn, centaury, leeks, and marjoram.

Gravel. - Butcher's-broom, ground-ivy, mallows, nettles, parsley, pennyroyal, horseradish, dandelion, burdock, pellitory-wall, marigolds, and medlars.

Gout. - Nettles, burdock, St. John's-wort, ground pine, crowfoot. This herb as an ointment melted with lard, buck-bean, and water dock of any kind.

Heart-burn. - Chamomile, saffron. Dose a drachm. Valerian, lovage, and water-cresses.

Hysterics. - Mother-wort, pennyroyal, pine, St. John's wort, valerain, southernwood, mugwort, and spear-mint.

Head-ache. - Primroses, holy thistle, sage, savory, thyme, sneeze-wort, vervain, cowslip, valerian-root; misletoe of the oak, rosemary,

Nervous Disorders. - Rosemary, sage, savory, thyme, valerian, vervain, cowslip, thyme, lily of the valley, celery, piony dwarf, and tormentil-root.

Piles. - Pile-wort, fig-wort, brook lime, mullein, toad-fax, lavender, comfrey, tormentil-root, shepherd's-purse.

To promote 'Perspiration. - Pine, viper's grass, pimpernell, elder flowers, borage, fumitory, and marigolds.

Scurvy. - Holy thistle, brook-lime, goose-grass, cresses, dandelion, endive, agrimony, lettuce, horse-radish, scurvy-grass, sorrel, succory, turnip, briony, water-dock, crowfoot, and fig-wort.

Spasms. - Lavender, mother-wort, peppermint, wood-betony, the lesser centaury.

RECIPES.

"He that would be long an old man must begin early to be one."
OLD AUTHOR.

A good Diet-drink for Meals. - Take half an ounce of ginger bruised, two ounces of bread toasted very brown, pour over it two quarts of boiling water, and stop it close. If this be done as soon as breakfast is over, it will be ready for dinner. It ought never to be drank colder than about eighty degrees, better known as blood heat.

Cholera. - Having received the three following receipts from a patient recently from India, I shall with much pleasure insert them. It is rather out of my course of practice; but I think they deserve a fair trial; and as the composition is such that it may be mixed and kept ready for use in every man's house, this information is deserving of notice. I have not proved their efficacy, but I confess I have a very high opinion of them.

The Indian Cure for the Cholera Morbus. One drachm of nitrous acid (not nitric), one ounce of peppermint-water or camphor mixture, and forty drops of tincture of opium. A fourth part of this mixture every three hours in a teacupful of gruel; the belly should be covered with a succession of hot cloths, and bottles of water applied to the feet.

Another. - Eighty drops of laudanum, wine-glass of brandy, and half a wine-glass of castor oil, mixed; if possible given at once, if not, one dessert spoonful after another until all is taken.

Another.-- A pill containing seven grains of calomel and one of opium. This may be repeated every hour until better.

Tilke's Pectoral Syrup. - This syrup is efficacious in asthmatic coughs and common colds. Even when the inflammation prevails, a teaspoonful morning, noon, and night, is a sufficient dose for grown persons. It may be given to children in small doses with perfect safety. This is worthy a fair trial. Price *2s. 9d.* and *4s. 6d.* per bottle.

To prevent Cramp. - Equal parts of salad oil and oil of rosemary; rub a little in with the band at bed-time on the calf of the leg, about three times a week.

A sure and easy Cure for the Piles. - One ounce of lenitive electuary, one ounce of milk of sulphur, one ounce of powder of gum arabic, half an ounce of cream of tartar, and as much syrup of violets as will make it into an electuary. A teaspoonful night and morning for nine successive days. To prevent the piles, take the same occasionally, and anoint the part with the fig leaf ointment. This may be depended on.

Ale for the inward Piles. Take one ounce of tormentil-root bruised, and boil it in a pint of good ale until reduced to half a pint; drink it blood-warm. Though a simple remedy, I have known this prove effectual when expensive medicines have failed.

For a Cough. - Oxymel of squills, syrup of poppies, and old rum, equal parts. One tea spoonful morning, noon, and night, in a wine-glass of sage or balm tea.

Another Way. - Three new-laid eggs, one ounce of honey, sweet-oil, lemon-juice, and old rum; beat them well together, then add half a pint of milk; stir it all one way. Dose a table-spoonful when the cough is troublesome.

For Weakness. One ounce of athea, (althea?) one ounce of mustard, one ounce cold-drawn oil, one ounce of honey, half an ounce balsam of Peru; mix. Take one teaspoonful morning and evening.

THE POOR MAN'S WEATHER-GLASS AND HUSBANDMAN'S BAROMETER.

Chickweed. - When the flower of this plant expands boldly in the morning, and continues open till twelve o'clock, no rain on that day; if it shuts, and covers the white flowers with its green mantle, the traveller had better take his great-coat and umbrella.

Pimpernell and Trefoil. - These plants fold up their leaves on the approach of rain.

Sowthistle. - If the flowers of this plant keep open all night it will be sure to rain next day. Good hint for those who go to Epsom races. Very interesting to watch this plant, how it turns towards the sun in the course of the day.

African Marygold. - If the flowers do not open by seven or eight in the morning, it will rain or thunder that day. Useful for those who keep Horses. - I have been a great admirer of that noble and useful animal the horse, which every day sets us an example; namely, to know when we have had enough both of eating and drinking; thus bringing to mind the old adage, that *"one may lead a horse to the river, but two cannot make him drink."*

I have been accustomed to keep two and sometimes three horses, for many years, and the great attachment which they exhibited towards me has often been remarked. Many of my friends observed that I could make them do every thing but speak. I sold a horse seven years since, now in my neighbourhood, and I think it would puzzle any one man to keep him from me if he heard my voice, without even seeing me. I will now with pleasure give the receipt, that others may enjoy the same gratification that I have:

Take one pound of oatmeal, a quarter pound of honey, a quarter pound of Spanish liquorice, half an ounce white briony in powder, one ounce of cuckoo pint in powder; mix all together and make a cake, bake it in a Dutch or other oven, carry it in your bosom for two or three days; fast your horse for a night and part of the day; then give him the cake out of your hand, broken in small pieces. If you repeat this occasionally he will never forget you, and you may do with him what no other person dare do. If you wish to see your horse always with a good coat (by the bye, this is necessary for us all), and to look superior to your neighbour's, give him the powder of white briony and cuckoo pint of each half an ounce in a small quantity of bran every day. It was by experiments on this noble animal that in a great measure I gained an insight into the cause and cure of disease; for a horse is much more delicate than a man. The first intimation my father had of my *penchant* was when I was nine years of age. He had a fixed day for horses to be brought for surgical operations, particularly that of *quittor*. On one occasion he was compelled to be at a neighbouring village, and left word that the horses, about three in number, should stop until his return. However I planned otherwise, and told the servants, if they would throw the horses on a bed of straw kept for that purpose, I would dress them. I did so, in a manner my father has many times said he could not improve on, But so determined was he that I should not follow this, or any medical pursuit, that he would never allow me to see him dress a horse afterwards, or let me get at any of his books. This so hurt my feelings, that at twelve years of age I left home, and at this tender age arrived in this great metropolis, a total stranger, and was obliged to follow the business I had been taught, although my mind soared to higher pursuits. The late Surgeon Heaviside, of George-street, Hanover-square, was the first who encouraged my partiality for the study of medicine; and although he is now gone

"To that bourne from whence no traveller returns,"

he still lives in my grateful memory. His kindness towards me (I was then fifteen) was that of a father. From that time to the present I have eagerly studied the cause of disease and the practice of medicine, purely for love of the pursuit, hardly anticipating the kind encouragement which I have so largely received from a liberal public.

LETTERS OF ACKNOWLEDGMENT

FOR THE

CURE OF GOUT, &c.

I SHALL now proceed to give a few of the numerous certificates I have had the satisfaction of receiving from some of those patients who have entrusted their lives in my hands. It is my practice to keep back the names of my patients, and the only exceptions I have made have been in those instances where the parties themselves have wished it, in order that their cases might bear the strongest corroboration. There is in many persons a natural reluctance to being placed too prominently before the public, especially those in an elevated sphere of life; I have therefore selected but very few letters, and generally those have been preferred, the writers of which have kindly stood forward in the vindication of my mode of treatment, and some who were themselves among the earliest that received cures at my hands.

In addition to these, I have selected several which refer more particularly to the accommodation and treatment they have received at my house. It is perhaps a pardonable vanity in me to refer particularly to these, as they convey useful information to the public, at the same time that they afford me the highest gratification. It may be considered something new, that persons undergoing processes to eradicate inveterate maladies, and this away from their homes, should speak of *comfort received*; but it is not the less true. I use very little restriction; my remedies act mildly and imperceptibly; the baths are a positive gratification; and, true it is, that surprise is invariably expressed by my in-door patients at the agreeable reception they experience.

To the Nobility and Gentry I am enabled to give personal reference to those in their own station of life, fully corroborating all that I have advanced. And the names of all parties alluded to in this work, will be readily supplied to every sincere inquirer after truth.

Among the following letters will be found one from Mr. COLEMAN, of No. 6, Westmoreland Street. I would refer inquirers to him particularly, being the first patient I attended and cured in a public capacity. His character, as a respectable tradesman, precludes the possibility of his being unduly biassed. For many years he was laid up for months at a time with the Gout, taken from his business, and put to an enormous expense for the best medical advice he could procure. He says truly, that in April 1830 he was suffering dreadfully with Gout, that he was speedily relieved, and that he has not since suffered one day from that complaint. He has called on me this month (Jan. 1834) in the best possible health, and will feel proud in giving every verbal explanation in his power; as well as refer to many others, whom he induced to partake of the same remedy on bearing of their infirmities.

The following is from a gentleman, who for a long period was beset with prejudices; but whose better judgment induced him to make a fair trial of what he was told concerning my practice. Personal reference will be given, in select cases:

Dear Sir: London, January 14th, 1834.

Accidently hearing of an enlarged edition of your Treatise on the Management of the Gout being in the press, will you have the goodness to direct your book seller to send me a dozen copies, as it will afford me great pleasure to recommend it to any afflicted friend.

From habits of early association, as well as family connection with members of the medical profession, perhaps few (if any) of your numerous patients could have felt greater reluctance than myself to have departed from the customary routine of the regular practitioner; but after occasional suffering for many years with Rheumatic Gout, without expectation of meeting with any permanent relief, I was agreeably surprised to find, under the blessing of Providence, your system completely adapted to my case, and that the domestic comforts of your establishment far exceeded my most sanguine expectation. Wishing your present work may be productive of a more extensive knowledge of the same,

I am, dear Sir, &c. &c. &c.

To Mr. Tilke, Thayer Street.

27, Goswell Terrace,
Goswell Road, Jan. 20, 1834.

Dear Sir:
Finding you have a book coming out and near completion, I take this early opportunity of expressing my approbation of your treatment, and wishing a few particulars of my case should be laid before the public; it was as follows:-Some weeks previous to my coming to you I caught cold, and was afterwards seized with what my medical adviser called the acute Rheumatism, (which was acute indeed!) the use of my limbs being entirely lost to me. After lingering a considerable time in a most painful state, and being reduced to a mere skeleton, the opinion of many friends being that I should not survive, I was induced by the recommendation of a gentleman to apply to you, and was brought to your house wrapt up in blankets, as my limbs were so painful and contracted I could not by any possibility rest. I am happy to state, from the assistance of your valuable medicated baths, and other most excellent remedies, I was enabled, after two days, to pace your house without assistance, and in one week to walk home with perfect ease and comfort, and am now perfectly restored to good health. I likewise have the gratification to believe you have removed a complaint in the chest, which I have suffered severely from for the last twelve years, during which time I have been under many of the faculty, including physicians. Dear Sir, if you think my case of sufficient importance for a space in your work, you are at perfect liberty to insert it.

I remain, Sir,
Yours respectfully,
HORATIO BARTLETT.

To Mr. TILKE, Thayer-street.

Near Lewes, Dec. 10th, 1833.

Sir:
I consider myself bound in gratitude to inform you that you have been the instrument of saving me from a severe fit of gout. You are aware, from my former letters, that the use of your medicines had kept off attacks, by using them as soon as I felt any symptoms. But being called from home suddenly the week before last, I had neglected to take your medicines with me. On the Tuesday morning my foot was stiff and rather painful, which symptoms increased through the day, and at night the pain was very severe. On Wednesday I returned home, and at night rubbed in the ointment on the feet, and took two of the gout pills. On Thursday morning the pain and inflammation were entirely gone, but the swelling remained. On Thursday and Friday nights I applied the ointment to the loins and chest, which I had not previously done; and the result was, that I was able to walk to church, and perform service both morning and afternoon, without any inconvenience to myself.

A little tenderness remained for a few days, but the ointment soon removed that also. As I think the efficacy of your remedies should be made well known, I beg you will make what use of this letter you please; and if you wish at any time to refer to me, you are at perfect liberty to do so; only, if you should in any future publication choose to insert this letter, I had rather my name should not be *printed*.

I am, Sir, your much obliged (Blank)
To Mr. Tilke.

(I have never had the pleasure of seeing this Reverend Gentleman, nor many others whose letters are in my possession.)

Tottenham-court Road, Dec. 8, 1833.

My dear Sir:

I have delayed writing to this period, almost doubting my own identity, being so entirely free from pain.

I think it a duty I owe to you and the public to state, that for the last nine or ten years I have been a great sufferer from the gout, the fits coming on so fast and severe, that I have been confined to my room for six months together, and at last was so much debilitated as to be quite unable to take any exercise, I heard of you by very accident, and determined to see you, although I confess I doubted your doing me any good, as I considered mine an almost hopeless case. I became your patient and inmate in February last, and I am happy to say I have been free from gout ever since, having had but one very slight attack, which I repelled in a few hours by following your instructions.

I am fully satisfied from my own experience that the gout is not (as it has been long thought) incurable; and those who are hard to believe, I would refer to Mr. Willis, of the Thatched House Tavern, St. James's street, who saw the dreadful state I was in when I became your patient. You are quite at liberty to give publicity to this, as I am anxious to bear testimony to the great benefit I have received from your treatment.

I am, dear Sir,
yours very truly,
J. HURD.

To Mr. Tilke, Thayer-street.

Sir;   Blackheath, Dec. 23, 1833.

It is with great satisfaction I am able to assure you that I have continued in perfect health since I left your house. I am the more anxious to acknowledge the benefit I have received at your hands, reflecting how great a sufferer I have been, and how little I expected more than perhaps a temporary relief when I first applied to you; and I must candidly say it was not with the most pleasurable feeling I left my home, uncertain as to what process I had to undergo when in your establishment, and you being an entire stranger to me. My surprise was great when I found myself in the midst of an agreeable family circle, and subjected to no tedious or harassing regimen, but partaking of the hospitality of a bountiful table, and the kind domestic attendance of Mrs. Tilke, at the same moment that my long-standing illness was being gradually undermined by your powerful Medicated Vapour Bath.

I think it but just to state thus much, as I consider myself highly indebted to you for a perfect state of health, and at the same time under an obligation for the very kind hospitality extended to me during the time I was under your roof.

I freely acknowledge the benefit and indulgences I have received from you and your family.

I remain your obliged friend,
W. WOODGATE.

Mr. Tilke, Thayer Street.

King's Head, Museum-street, Jan. 1, 1834.

Dear Sir;

I beg leave to address you with feelings of gratitude and admiration for the attention and skill you have bestowed upon my case; and I now take the earliest opportunity of expressing my sense of the kind and humane treatment I have received at your hands, and to acknowledge the superior efficacy of your medicines. I had been afflicted with the gout for the last twenty years, and had frequently been incapacitated for several months together from attending to my business; the paroxysms of my complaint were severe, and the repeated shocks it had given to my constitution had made me almost despair of ever discovering an antidote for my sufferings, until strongly recommended by the medical gentleman who had attended me for years, and who could afford me little or no relief (although highly eminent in his profession) to try your baths and medicine, which I am most happy to say have proved in every respect quite successful; so much so, that I am perfectly recovered, and am at this moment enjoying better health than I have for years.

I cannot allow this opportunity to escape without returning my best thank to Mrs. Tilke, for her very kind attentions to me during my stay with you.

You have my permission to make this as public as possible, and beg leave to add, that I shall be most happy to explain to any one the superior advantages of your treatment of the gout.

I am, dear Sir, yours truly,
J. FELLOW.

Mr. S. W. Tilke, Thayer-street.

76, Long-Acre, 1st January 1834.

Dear Sir; I have great satisfaction in acknowledging the benefit I have received from your treatment of the rheumatism, with which disease I have been for some years afflicted, and for which I have sought relief by vapour baths, on the Continent and in Turkey; and it is due to you to state that I have received so much benefit from your vapour baths, ointment, and pills, in eight days, that I am now relieved from the most excruciating pains.

I beg at the same time to notice, that I consider your vapour baths superior and more effectual than any I have ever had either in England or abroad; and I shall certainly take every opportunity of making this known, as well as the constant kind attention which is paid to the comfort of the patients under your care. It should be very generally known, for the sake of invalids afflicted with gout or rheumatism, or others who occasionally take baths, that such a pleasant retreat is to be found in the midst of your most excellent family.

I am, dear Sir,

most faithfully yours,

THOMAS BARRETT.

To Mr. Tilke, No. 8, Thayer-street, Manchester-square.

Extract of a Letter from a Lady after residing in my house as a patient. - *"Permit me to add, that not the least among the strange things you have accomplished, is the curing of a laudanum-taker of the habit of using that deadly drug every night for five years. Thank heaven and you I have conquered it, and nothing shall induce me ever to have recourse to it again. I assure you no opportunity shall be omitted in advising sufferers to obtain similar benefits to what I have in mercy received."*

Extract of a private Letter received from a Gentleman of Cambridge, speaking of a Reverend Gentleman whom he had recommended to me. - *"I have great pleasure in informing you that your medicine has been decidedly successful in the case of the Rev. (Blank) of (Blank), whom I recommended three months ago; indeed, he is so confident of its effects, that on Whit-Monday I met him at a public dinner, when the moment he saw me he rose from the table, and before the company thanked me for having recommended a medicine which has cured him of a disorder (the gout,) hitherto considered incurable."*

No. 1, St. John's Square, Clerkenwell,
February 4th, 1832.

Dear Sir: -Understanding you are about publishing a little work on the nature of the Gout and Ringworm, I beg, for the sake of the Public as well as yourself, to offer you my opinion upon your treatment of the former, hoping you will publish it in your book, as it may fall under the observation of many who know what I have suffered. I have been upwards of twenty years much afflicted with the Gout; have been in many parts of the world; have tried all remedies, both at home and abroad, and not until I put myself under your care (about six months since) did I ever experience so much benefit.

Your powders and ointment I do consider to be the best medicine ever yet discovered for the gout; and if you possess the same knowledge of the ringworm, it certainly must be considered of great national importance. Feeling grateful for your great attention to me, since I have been under your care, I beg to say, I shall always be happy in explaining to any persons, you may think proper to refer to me. I am, dear Sir, your obliged and humble servant WM. HOAR.

To Mr. Tilke, 8, Thayer Street.

14, York Buildings, New Road,

February 5th, 1832.

Dear Sir: - In November last I had a most violent attack of the Rheumatic Gout over my limbs, which confined me to my bed. On these occasions I experience the most excruciating pains, having been severely afflicted for the last twelve years, brought on, I believe, from my campaigns with the Duke of Wellington in the Peninsula. Knowing you had attended several of my friends, and been successful in all cases, by their strict attention to the use of your ointment, I resolved to have recourse to the same; and being satisfied that your system of rubbing does not cause any excoriation, I allowed a trial, and to my utter astonishment, within twelve hours after your (truly named infallible) ointment had been applied, all symptoms of gout have vanished; and I have not since had the slightest return of gout. I have written this letter, that you may lay it before the public, if you see proper. In thus doing, I feel that I am discharging a duty which I owe, as well to the public as to yourself.

I am, Sir, yours very respectfully,

EDWARD HODGES.

To Mr. Tilke, Thayer Street.

204 Regent Street, London, Feb. 2d, 1832.

Dear Sir -In justice to you, and from a sense of feeling to my fellow sufferers who may be afflicted with that dreadful malady the Gout, I am happy to bear testimony to the safety and certainty of a cure performed on me by following your prescriptions and directions, and which has been effected in a much shorter time than I expected. About eight months back I had a very severe attack of the Gout, which rendered me almost helpless; but after four days' adherence to your directions I have, thank God, quite recovered the use of my limbs, and am now quite well. I am also very happy to bear testimony to the extraordinary, and indeed almost unexpected cure which you performed on Mr. Newman.

Hoping your exertions may meet that reward which they so justly merit, and which in my opinion require only to be known to be fully appreciated,

I am, dear Sir, your obedient servant,

R. HUNTLEY .

To Mr. Tilke, 8, Thayer Street.

Howland Street, February 4th, 1832.

Dear Sir; -With pleasure I transmit you a few lines, stating in a very limited degree the effect your valuable Ointment has had on me.

I have been a great sufferer for nineteen years, some years confined for four months out of the twelve; and about three years since I was three months from my business with the Gout. It would be impossible for me to enumerate the many different medicines (strongly recommended for Gout) I have used; also the various other applications tried, such as fomentations, poultices, leeches, &c. without any real benefit.

About eighteen months since I was attacked with a severe fit of Gout, and the paroxysm was very acute for two nights. I desired some of my family to send for your Ointment, and I must confess I joined with them in thinking I should not receive much benefit from the use of it. However, when brought it was well rubbed in, and again in the afternoon. My sufferings after the second rubbing were very great for a few hours, after which time pimples made their appearance; and from that period, with gratitude I state it to you as the instrument, I have had but very little pain from gout. I do not mean to infer that I have not had any gout or pain since that time; yet I do say that my pain has not been worth mentioning, to that which I formerly endured.

I further state, my limbs are much stronger; also my general health is much improved; so much so, that I have been enabled to take a more active part in my business the last six months than I did during the last five years.

If you think well to make this letter public, I wish most explicitly to state, that it would be useless for any one to expect benefit from your ointment unless they tenaciously adhere to your directions. I would just add, that I much approve of your Powders.

Wishing you, my dear Sir, health and prosperity, I remain,

Your's very truly,

J. SWEETLAND.

To Mr. Tilke, Thayer Street.

Old Cavendish Street, Sept 14, 1831.

Sir;-For the last twenty years I have been subject to attacks of Gout, every year the complaint increasing; so much so, that the last attack before I sent for you (which was last February) confined me to my room sixteen weeks. I was then advised to send for you. I followed the directions laid down, and in a week was enabled to leave my room; since which time I have had no return of the complaint of any consequence but what a few of the powders and once or twice applying the ointment will remove. My general health is improved from the efficacy of the powders and ointment.

I am, Sir, your's respectfully,

To Mr. Tilke, Thayer Street.   R. NEWMAN.

P.S. I have recommended several of my friends, who have found great benefit from the application and powders; and I shall be happy to explain to any person the benefit I have received.

Extract of a Private Letter from a Reverend Gentleman who had suffered many years with attacks of Gout.

January 4th 1831.

Sir; -I beg to inform you that I have derived great benefit from your Gout Ointment, as far as regards attacks in the joints, as it certainly removes it with much greater certainty and safety than any internal remedies; and I would also state, that it strengthens the limbs, and prevents that painful stiffness and weakness which I have suffered so much from after being exposed to cold and damp.

2, Silver Street, Clerkenwell, Feb. 2, 1832.

Dear Sir; -I wish to add my testimony to the efficacy of your valuable Gout Medicine, having received a great benefit from it. I have been troubled with the Gout many years, and last summer I had it eight weeks. Complaining to a friend of the pain I was suffering, and great inconvenience in my business, he recommended me to try your Ointment, which had done Captain Hoar, of St. John's Square, so much good.   I did so; and the result was, on the third day I walked five miles without inconvenience; nor have I any fear except from my own neglect, in not attending to your directions.

I am, Sir, your's very truly,

G. CHAPPEIL.

To Mr. Tilke, Thayer Street

No. 6, Westmoreland Street, Mary-le-bone, August 10th, 1830.

Dear Sir; -Having had, in the beginning of April last, a severe attack of Rheumatic Gout in my legs and feet, so much so as totally to deprive me of the use of them, and suffering the most excruciating pain for several days, being confined to my bed, a friend came to see me, and strongly recommended your Ointment, a pot of which he brought with him, stating it was an infallible cure. The inflammation and swelling in my limbs at this time was very great, and the pain intense, and being most anxious for relief, I had the ointment applied to the parts affected, when to my astonishment, in a short time after the rubbing the pain ceased, in the course of the night the swelling abated, and the following day I was able to walk about my bed-room, comparatively free from the complaint.

Now, Sir, as I have been a great martyr to the Rheumatic Gout before, and been under some of the most eminent of the Faculty for three and four months at a time, I consider I should not do you justice without thus publicly making it known, and beg you will make use of this letter in any way you see proper, for the benefit of mankind.

I am, Sir, your's very truly,

To Mr. Tilke, Thayer-street.   T. COLEMAN.

P.S. I have just learnt that you are about publishing a few remarks on your method of treating the Gout. If it is intended to publish my letter, it is my wish that the following fact may be added in a Postscript, *viz.* that although eighteen months have elapsed since it was written, I have remained free from any serious attack of gout, and my general health is altogether improved. I have several times felt slight symptoms of the complaint after having caught cold; but on having recourse to the ointment, this has been instantly removed. In consequence of the very great benefit I have received, I have in many instances induced my friends who have been suffering from the same complaint to try the same remedy, and it has invariably succeeded up to the present period, February 25th, 1832.

No. 23, Bowling Green Lane, Clerkenwell,
July 30th, 1830.

Dear Sir: -I trust you will excuse the liberty I take in addressing you, but the benefit I have received from the Use of your Rheumatic Ointment induces me to make my case known to you (and likewise the public, should you think proper). I have been afflicted for the last twelve-months with a severe rheumatic affection in my head and neck, which completely prevented me from following my business; in fact, I could not turn my head and neck without at the same time turning my body, and the pain was so excessive day and night, that I was never at ease for one hour. After being under an eminent physician for several months without receiving any benefit, I was advised to try Middlesex Hospital, where I was an out-patient for two months, but still without receiving any benefit. At length a friend by great persuasion, prevailed upon me to try your ointment, and after attending to the directions given for three weeks, the pains in my head left me, and I could move my neck with the greatest facility, and in a few days after I was able to pursue my business. I shall at all times be extremely happy to give every information in my power to persons similarly afflicted, who may call upon me, and with the hope that the good effects of the ointment may be known in every part of the world,

I remain, Sir, with respect, your obliged servant,
G. BRADWITH.

To Mr. Tilke, Thayer Street.

No. 5, Charles Street, Lisson Green,
25th Septemher, 1830.

Dear Sir: -At the commencement of last month I had a violent attack of the Rheumatic Gout over the whole of my limbs, which confined me so closely to my bed that it was impossible for me to stand at all without assistance; on such occasions I experienced the most excruciating pains. For above six weeks I was most bitterly tortured, notwithstanding I was attended by some of the first medical practitioners in this country. After this period I was induced, by the persuasion of my friends, to use your (properly named infallible) ointment; and after using between two and three pots, I recovered so as to be able to walk; and in less than a week all pain, swelling, and inflammation were entirely removed. I think I am doing but an act of justice, both to yourself and the public, in thus publicly stating the particulars of the astonishingly rapid cure performed on me by your ointment, and I beg you to give what publicity you please to this letter.

I am, Sir, with thanks and gratitude, your's obediently,

To Mr. Tilke, Thayer Street.
M. BARKER.

No. 1, High Street, Mary-le -bone,
February 16th, 1831.

Dear Sir:-After having delayed writing for four months since my last fit of the Gout, that I might prove the real efficacy of your (I have reason to say) invaluable Gout Ointment, I beg leave now to give you some account of its effects and mode of operating on me.

When I first began to use the Ointment I had been subject to Gout twelve years, having three or four severe fits every year, and was then suffering under a *very severe one*. The first pot produced no other effect than very considerably increasing the pain . I still determined on persevering, and on using the second pot my feet were quickly covered with pimples filled with a watery matter, and itching much, but occasioning no pain; after which I got well rapidly. Upon the second attack the effects were the same, but the fit much shorter. The last time I had it in hands and feet, but the fit was still shorter; since which I have known nothing of gout, for on feeling any symptoms, I invariably bathe my feet and hands in warm water, and rub in the ointment on going to bed; the following morning I feel no more of it. I ought per haps to say it is my opinion the goutic matter is extracted, and the joints and feet strengthened, by the ointment. I have been thus particular as I wish you to make what use you can of this, for the information and benefit of others, who may be afflicted as I have been.

I am, dear Sir, your's very truly,

To Mr. Tilke, Thayer Street.
J.L. KEEBLE .

Sir: - I trouble you with this short letter to inform you, that from the time of using your Ointment, in September 1830, to the present moment, I have been entirely free from all return of that severe complaint. I am desirous of your being aware of this fact, as it will serve to shew that the cure, while it was rapid, is also of the most effectual nature. -M. B. January 10, 1834.

February, 1831.

Dear Sir; -As I have recently witnessed a surprisingly rapid cure of Rheumatic Gout in my family by the application of your Ointment, I feel I am performing a duty to you, as well as the public, in detailing the following facts. In the latter end of January one of my family was seized with violent pains in the limbs, which became swelled and inflamed, with all the distressing accompaniments of the severest Rheumatic Gout. Previous to this I had known of a most rapid cure performed by your ointment, in the case of a niece of mine, who had caught cold, and suffered greatly in all her limbs (but which pains were removed as by magic when your ointment was applied), and knowing of many other cures equally surprising, I hesitated not a moment in ordering your ointment to my own daughter. It was not at first possible to rub in the ointment, from the pain it caused, it was therefore spread on till the pain abated, and afterwards well and frequently rubbed in. Now, Sir, mark what follows, the truth of which I solemnly aver. The pain was removed in four-and-twenty hours; the swelling gradually abated, the use of the limbs in a few days recovered, and within twelve days of the first attack she was able to attend an evening party, and danced several hours. I have only to add, Sir, that the truth of the above will be substantiated by myself at any time you may require it; and I am of opinion that persons labouring under this or similar complaints, knowing of your very simple remedy, and not availing themselves of it, may be henceforward considered voluntary sufferers.

I remain, my dear Sir, yours very truly,

J. P.

ON THE

NATURE AND TREATMENT

OF

SCALLED HEAD AND RING -WORM.

"After we have practised good actions awhile, they become easy; and when they are easy, we begin to take pleasure in them; and when they please us, we do them frequently; and by frequency of acts a thing grows into habit, and confirmed habit is a kind of second nature; and so far as any thing is natural, so far it is necessary, and we can hardly do otherwise; nay, we do it many times when we do not think of it."

ARCHBISHOP TILLOTSON.

SCALLED HEAD,

OR, "Tinea Capitis," as the gentlemen of the Medical Profession term it, is a disease of a most malignant and contagious nature, and melancholy to relate, is spreading far, and making most rapid progress throughout the kingdom; a circumstance which makes it a consideration of vast importance to those who have the care of children, or, in other words, who keep schools; to those it has always been a subject of dread, from the known fact of its being contagious, and the means of cure, as far as generally known, very uncertain and dilatory. Bonetus says, *"There are no proper and certain remedies yet found out for the cure of this stubborn distemper."* Another author advises us not to be over hasty in attempting to cure this disorder, *"unless the adjacent parts are in danger of being injured."* How often have I, within the last ten years, witnessed the dreadful havoc of this disease on the constitution! Many children have been brought to me, after suffering for four and five years, until the disease has proved most destructive to them, not unlike the rot in sheep, passing down the chest and back. I have often been compelled to fasten up their ears with a bandage, to prevent their hanging down.

Next to the disease of which I have been speaking in the former part of this little pamphlet, perhaps none is more difficult to cure, or any that so strongly opposes almost every attempt of the professional man. Independently of this, it is marked for its peculiar and perplexing character, in defying any one general and steady system of practice, inasmuch as that, according to ordinary means, if, I will say, twenty children are selected, each of the same age, and each afflicted with this disease, of about the same standing and appearance, scarce any single remedy that would cure one would be of the least service to the other; so that you must begin your plan of treatment with twenty different remedies, and change these remedies, perhaps, fifty times, and after all, leave off as bad, or worse, than when you began.

The seat of this disease is on the head, and the victims of it are generally children of tender age; it commences by forming little ulcers in and about the bulbs where the hair takes root; these bursting, pour out a matter, which being blended with the natural moisture and even filth of the surrounding parts, and exposed to the influence of the atmosphere, becomes of a most disagreeable, filthy, offensive, and acrid nature; it then generally collects into and forms large scabs over the surface of the head, which continually break, crack, or peel off, leaving the poor sufferer the object of disgust with many, while the feelings of others must be aroused to the greatest commiseration. When this disease has continued for some time, resisting every attempt at cure, it arrives at the utmost degree of inveteracy, and the matter poured out by it becomes absorbed and taken up into the system, and the whole mass of blood being impregnated with it, it breaks out into innumerable forms of disease; sometimes glandular swellings in various parts of the body, at other times by eruptive pimples, pains and aches in the bones, swellings at the large joint, fevers, loss of appetite, general wasting, and death. While writing this I have just had a young lady, about fifteen, placed under my care for the above disease; a letter accompanied her to me from her mother, wherein she says: - *"We are quite uneasy about it, for we have lost a fine little boy with the Scalled head."* The letter may be seen. It will be here necessary to explain, that Scalled-head is often mistaken for a disease of a more simple kind, as when a few pimples appear in consequence of some interruption that has probably taken place from obstruction in the pores, or some other trifling cause. I therefore warn all parents not to trust to their own judgment in these matters, as they may often be led to use dangerous and improper remedies, that would even aggravate these little pimples into more extensive and dangerous maladies.

Perhaps there is no disease more dependent on Cleanliness than Scalled-head; in deed, under no treatment can success be expected without a steady attention to this part of the curative process; and to facilitate this the more, as soon as the disease is discovered, the hair should be all cut off, the head then shaved, and carefully washed with warm water; having effected this, it is all that the parent or nurse should attempt to do; beyond this, be assured, such is the nature of the disease, that every domestic attempt at cure is attended with the most dangerous consequences, even to the life of the sufferer.

Many are the remedies in fashion for at tempting to cure this malady; such as muriatic acid, sulphur, tar, turpentine, blisters, ointments, and that barbarous treatment of pulling the hairs out of the head by the root, &c.; but the most to be dreaded, is the free and unrestrained use of mercury, which is often pushed in the most violent and virulent forms, to the most fearful and frightful extremes, as is often to be traced in the sad and incurable malady of water on the brain, honey-combed skull; not unfrequently the total loss of sight; and lastly, death itself.

Thus the remedies are rendered as alarming, and even more to be dreaded than the disease.

It is presumed, that the obstinacy of this disease, as well as the fact of its being extremely contagious, are generally known to the public; but are they as well aware, that to the present moment there is no such thing as a certain cure to be met with, beyond what I myself practise? To put this in a more clear point of view, I shall point to the School of Christ's Hospital, better known as "the Blue-Coat School," which, I believe, has had this complaint, more or less, for nine years in succession; although it can not be doubted, they have had recourse to the first medical advice. Less than three years since the subject was brought more particularly to my notice by a letter in the 'Times', in reply to the complaints of many parents of the pupils, that their children were delayed considerably beyond the usual period at the preparatory school at Hertford. This letter candidly stated, that the only reason for the great delay was, that they were desirous of not introducing the Ringworm into the London school, as it was very prevalent in the school at Hertford. No doubt this excellent institution has funds to command the best advice to be found in Europe; and yet the complaint has existed there for years. This too plainly shews, what I believe has been very generally admitted by medical men, that a certain remedy is not known.

In the course of the two last years I have had several children of this school brought to me by their parents, hoping, yet doubting whether it were possible that I could do any good, where so much had before been tried in vain. In all these cases perfect cures were performed, and the parents are most anxious to corroborate the efficacy of them. I

now publicly announce to the Governors and conductors of all public institutions, that I will take the whole, or any number of the worst cases to be met with in any establishment, and undertake the cure, and if I fail in the attempt, the loss shall be my own. The more public the ordeal before which this might be performed, the more would it be to my satisfaction.

It surely will be unpardonable, after this public announcement, if the Governors of establishments will any longer allow this disease to exist, where the cure is so certain. If the truth of what I have stated be doubted, let the most sceptical call on me, and I will give them ocular proof of daily cures I am performing.

In more than one instance it has happened, that Proprietors of Schools have come to me in the greatest anxiety of mind, alarmed at the rapid spread of this complaint in their establishments, and stating that their prospects would be ruined if means were not discovered to arrest its progress. It was with the greatest feelings of satisfaction that I took these formidable cases in hand, and the complaint has been actually removed, without even the scholars themselves being aware of the situation in which they stood, and the feelings of their parents spared from unavailing anxiety. The names of persons and places have been held back from obvious motives, and although I have here stated the general facts, nothing will ever induce me to name the parties thus circumstanced without their permission.

It only remains for me to add, after these few remarks, that I have for many years employed a vegetable system of cure for this direful scourge; simple in its nature, certain in its effects, free from injury, and generally rapid in its cure, and I am happy in being enabled to say, that I not only possess the remedy, but that I have been blessed with, during a lengthened practice, hundreds of successful cases, for never up to this moment have I failed in one. References can be given to many a glad father, many a thankful mother, and to many a heart of gratitude in young people, for the cures which I have performed, independently of very many medical men, who have turned over their patients to my care, after every effort and ineffectual attempt to stop its rapid career. And proud am I to say too, that I have at this moment the children of several highly distinguished professional gentlemen under my entire management.

My peculiar mode of practice consists in many different modes of treatment, according to the constitution, age, sex, nature, and appearance of the disease in different patients. With some after many months, or after years standing, I give a botanic vapour-bath to the *head only* (for the performance of which I have invented a little apparatus); as this in dry, scorbutic cases, opens the pores of the skin, and the more readily admits my ointment; the power of which expels all offensive matter from the head, and I am often obliged to have the assistance of my Gout Ointment applied to the Chest; which with my Powders soon sets the blood in free circulation, by which means, or by a sort of gentle *Perspiration*, some of the impure fluid or matter is thrown off by the pores of the skin. I am now speaking of the worst species; and I think there are about nine different sorts. Some require my Ringworm Ointment alone, or the assistance of my herb tea, which I often give. I have just effected a cure of six children in one family. The mother informed me her eldest daughter brought it from school, and gave it to the other five children; not two of them had the same disease, and I was obliged to use different means with each child. I am sure medical gentlemen will believe this part of my statement, as it forms the difficulty in the cure of the disease, which they cannot conquer or explain.

LETTERS.

The following letter was received from a Member of Parliament, acknowledging the cure of his son.

27th Jan. 1832.

Sir: -- I feel great pleasure in bearing testimony to your skill in the treatment of Ring-worm. About two years ago, my eldest son, then between nine and ten years of age, returned from school, where he had contracted the above disease. For upwards of nine months he was under many hands, medical and non-medical, without experiencing the least benefit. Recommended to you, after three dressings only, in less than one month he was perfectly cured. I consider your knowledge and treatment to be of great public importance, and I remain, Sir, your's obediently,

W. M.

To Mr. Tilke, 8, Thayer-street.

17, Vere Street, Cavendish Square, Jan, 27th, 1832.

Dear Sir: - I have been anxious, for some time, to acknowledge the benefit which my little boy experienced from your treatment of the Ring-worm, which you may probably recollect you cured about twelve months ago. I had tried many highly respectable gentlemen of the faculty, without making the smallest progress towards amendment, for upwards of six months. Under your treatment, every vestige of disease disappeared in less than three weeks. I should have expressed my gratitude before this, but waited to ascertain if any eruption should appear, and have now great pleasure in stating to you that his head continues perfectly clean, without the smallest appearance of scurf.

I am, dear Sir, with much respect, your obedient servant,

CHARLES BIRCH,

To Mr. Tilke, Thayer Street.

24, Bentinck Street, Cavendish Square, Feb. 13th 1832.

Dear Sir: -- I feel it my incumbent duty, both to you and the public, to acknowledge the cure of the Scalled Head which you performed upon my little boy about nine years of age, he having been treated for it at school, where he had been for some months, with the appearance of the disease getting obviously worse, up to the time of your treatment, to which, I am happy to say, it immediately yielded, and was cured in the course of three weeks, and the hair brought over the head. This cannot but be viewed as of great consequence to the public at large, as your mode of treatment has for its object the cleansing impurities out of the system, both in this as well as the Ring-Worm, which I find from my friends you treat with equal success: a circumstance that I hope, for the good of the rising generation, may not be overlooked, as it has, unfortunately, in some of our large schools, been done for the last two years.

I am, Sir, your's truly,

W. H. BAYLY.

To Mr. Tilke, 8, Thayer Street.

36, Lamb's Conduit Street, 7th Feb. 1832.

Sir: -I feel anxious to bear my testimony to the success of your treatment of Ring-Worm. About eighteen months ago, my eldest son, now seven years of age, contracted the above disease at school, and for six months we had recourse to the best advice, without experiencing the least benefit. You were recommended to me by Mr. Hollis, and the child brought to you. After two or three dressings, in less than a month we perceived the worm cured, and dying away. I had another son, exactly the same, but under no one's hands but your own; his you cured in a very short time, I think in about a fortnight or three weeks. We also had a niece, who came from school with a very obstinate disease; you cured the child's head, to the amazement and surprise of her friends; for it had been so long incurable and badly treated, that part of the child's head was burnt in white spots, and now the hair will never grow on those places where they were so dreadfully treated. I consider your know ledge of this disease to be of great public benefit.

I remain, Sir, yours, &c.

To Mr. Tilke, 8, Thayer Street.   J. B. Pain

10, Cleveland Street, Fitzroy Square, Feb. 7th, 1832.

Sir: -- I have a son who had contracted that very troublesome disorder, the Ring-Worm, which he retained nearly two years, during which time he was attended by three medical gentlemen, without deriving any apparent benefit. Fortunately I met a friend who assured me you had cured some of his family, which induced me to make a trial of your skill, and to my great joy, I found that in one week the complaint was quite removed. It is full a twelvemonth since the cure has been made, and no symptom of return has appeared.

I remain, Sir, your's most respectfully,

To Mr. Tilke, 8, Thayer-street.   J. Hollis.

No. 1, North Street, January 1832.

Dear Sir:-Gratitude prompts me to return you my humble thanks for the effectual cure of my daughter with that most distressing malady, the Scalled-Head. Twelve months have now elapsed, and there are no signs of any return. Mrs. Smith joins me in wishing you every success your discovery merits.

I remain, dear Sir, your most obedient servant,

To Mr. Tilke, 8, Thayer Street.   FREDERICK SMITH.

46, Great Mary-le- bone Street, Feb. 6, 1832.

Sir: -I think it but right that I should let you know how grateful I feel for the cure of my son of the Ring Worm. I tried many prescriptions without the least avail, until hearing of your medicine, which by being applied three times has entirely cured him.

I remain, your obedient servant,

To Mr. Tilke, 8, Thayer Street.   J. BATCHELOR.

85, Edgeware Road, Feb. 18, 1832.

Dear Sir: – You will no doubt be surprised at my writing this, never having had the pleasure of seeing you; but the wish I have of giving publicity, by every means in my power, to your treatment of that very troublesome disease called Scalled-head, has induced me to take this course; that you may both show this, and refer any patients to me (if you think proper), who have children with the same complaint. The result of your treatment must be of the utmost importance to parents.

Last June my child was attacked with this complaint, who was then put under the care of our doctor, who tried every means he could think of for three months, without the least advantage. He then recommended sea air, and she was sent to Ramsgate for a month; but came back worse, if possible. - We then had recourse to various applications with as little success; till hearing of a family of six children who were cured by you, I agreed to put her under your care, when in the short space of four weeks she perfectly recovered. You not having before known the whole of this case, could hardly conceive the gratitude and pleasure we have experienced in her recovery. Again wishing you make use of this in any way you think proper for the relief of those afflicted with this most obstinate disease,

I subscribe myself, your's most respectfully,

To Mr. Tilke, 8, Thayer Street.   W. HAYNES.

No. 96, Cheapside, Feb. 29, 1832.

Dear Sir: -I must apologize for what may appear a neglect in not answering your kind inquiries respecting the health of my children, by referring you to my recent domestic calamity as the sole cause. As respects my children, however severe and desperate one of their cases of Ringworm was, I am happy to inform you they appear equally cured; the severer case of the two only now requiring a little extra attention from the rising of the scurf; and I beg sincerely to assure you, that in my estimation a parent's gratitude must be added to the trivial expense of your ointment and kind attention, and which alone can render an equivalent for the extraordinary and rapid cure you have effected, particularly when I place it in comparison with the great expense, anxiety, and trouble I and my family have been at and endured, during the time they were under the care of several of the faculty, for upwards of two years before I was providentially recommended to you. Permit me to add, that I shall be most happy to shew the children to any person you may refer to me, or answer any inquiries; and I feel it an incumbent duty towards other parents to request you will make use of this testimony, in any way you may think best, to promote the publicity of your invaluable remedy.

Believe me, dear Sir, to remain your's ever obliged,

To Mr. Tilke, Thayer Street.   W. TURNER.

73, Strand, March 2 , 1832.

Dear Sir: - I beg to return you my best thanks for the kind care and attention my little boy has experienced from you, having been some time afflicted with that very unpleasant disorder the Scalled-Head; and I have great pleasure in saying, that I have every reason to think a perfect cure has been effected.

I am, dear Sir, your obliged servant,

To Mr. Tilke, Thayer Street.   WM. TATE.

"Will Fortune never come with both hands full?
She either gives a Stomach and no food, (Such are the poor in health); or else a feast,
And takes away the Stomach, (such are the rich,
That have abundance, and enjoy it not.)".

"If the Cook make the Gluttony,
She helps to make the Disease."
SHAKSPEARE.

ON SCARLET FEVER.

"To prevent diseases is surely a more advantageous art to mankind than to cure them. But the sagacity to comprehend and estimate the importance of uncontemplated improvement, is confined to a very few, on whom Nature has bestowed a sufficient degree of perfection of the sense, which is to measure it; the candour to make a fair report of it is still more uncommon; it cannot often be expected from those whose most vital interest it is to prevent the development of that by which their own importance, perhaps their only means of existence, may be for ever eclipsed." - Dr. KITCHENER.

Dr. Starke says, "The only test of the utility of knowledge is its promoting the happiness of mankind."

FIELDING has said, in some part of his works, that when a man commences writing a book, circumstances during his labour may occur to lead him into matter which he had no intention of touching on. Domestic calamity has most acutely shewn the application of this remark to myself, and made me feel that

"Every one can master grief
But he that has it."
SHAKSPEARE.

The Scarlet Fever raged in my family; I had recourse to medical men, whose practice, no doubt, was regulated according to the rules laid down for their guide; and, in the end, I have to lament the loss of a dear daughter and sister. I do consider that the treatment was contrary to nature. I would by no means wish to deter my readers from the exercise of their own judgments; I only wish to communicate what I consider an easy, and I have no doubt successful method of treatment; for I hold that the man who feels dissatisfied with what he sees in practice, and takes up his pen, and boldly gives to the world his opinions, is more to be praised than he who in private society, with a deceptive smile, *"just hints a fault, and hesitates dislike."*

It will, no doubt, excite surprise in some, that I should have called in advice which I had so little confidence in; but it must be remembered, that it is not customary in the medical profession to prescribe for your own family; and every one will readily see the necessity there is for me to be careful to give no pretence to cavillers. Besides,

> "I can easier teach twenty
> What were good to be done,
> Than be one of the twenty
> To follow mine own teaching."
> SHAKSPEARE.

That eminent man, Dr. Clark, has told us, that *"the loss of one practical fact is a robbery on the public. It is incumbent on everyone to throw his mite into the mass; indeed, it is doubtful how a man can answer to his conscience having indolently deprived the world of that which, if communicated, might have added to the safety of a fellow-creature."* Believing all this firmly as I do, I should not be doing my duty to the public, if I were not to give my opinion as to the treatment and cure of this disease.

I believe, if the efforts of nature, in the beginning of a fever, were duly attended to, and promoted, it would seldom be attended with danger; but when they are either neglected or counteracted, it is no wonder if the disease proves fatal. Persons residing in the country have a common, and I believe a very just notion, that sweating is necessary in fever, as all fevers proceed from an obstructed perspiration. The French are of the same opinion, as they seldom give any other medicine than elder flowers in an infusion, and put warm bladders of water to the feet. Perspiration follows, the pores of the skin are opened, by which means the fever is carried off, as all fevers are only an effort of nature to free herself from an offending cause; and, indeed, those who have the lives of their fellow-men placed in their hands, ought to be taught and well observe what means nature takes, unassisted by art, to relieve herself from these diseased humours. Many important hints from the above may be taken, and those who would advance and improve the study of the healing art, ought to rest satisfied with a few but well-chosen medicines for each disease, and be rightly acquainted with their power and efficacy in different constitutions; they should despise the cumbersome load of applications such as modern practice abounds in, and the use of which too often proves fatal. I offer the following suggestions, to show my readers how they may with safety treat patients with the Scarlet Fever; being the course I shall pursue, should I be so unfortunate as to have any more of my family affected with this distemper. Common sense points out to us that it must be proper and safe, although contrary to the common practice of the day.

Scarlet Fever derived its name from the colour of the skin, more particularly on the joints, which appear as if coloured with red wine. It begins with a sore throat, and, like other fevers, with coldness and shiverings. The colour on the skin will disappear on the third or fourth day, if improperly treated with bleeding and cold applications, in which case it is always dangerous, as this is attended, first, with languor, sickness, and great oppression, and much heat; quick pulse, but small and depressed, the breathing short and laborious, the skin hot and dry, the tongue moist and covered with a whitish mucus, costiveness, and retention of urine. As these symptoms, if not removed, must prove fatal in a few days, they require the promptest applications. There is no disease where the steam bath, charged with fumitory and hops, may be used with more apparent success than this, as it is attended with a soothing and composing effect, and induces refreshing sleep, and by relaxing the surface, perspiration is easily attained. From this cause a steam-bath must be serviceable in fevers, both in soliciting the fluids to the skin, and by the cooling process of evaporation, which abates the extreme heat, and mitigates the feverish condition; and the venom of this disease, which has produced the danger before-named, will be expelled through the pores of the skin. Assist this by giving the following expulsive medicine:

Of elder-flowers, of fumitory, and of borage, each half-an-ounce, with five grains of saffron-leaf, boiled in one quart of milk for about ten minutes. Let one-fourth of this be taken every hour, unless the perspiration be very great, when half the quantity may do. If there is an inclination to vomit, give an infusion of green tea and one grain of tartar emetic with it, or three grains of ipecacuanha in a little warm water. This may be repeated in one hour, should there be no effect. The throat may be gargled with sage, vinegar and honey, boiled together, and the steam from this may be conveyed to the throat through a funnel by the mouth. After the violence of the disease is over, the body should be kept open with mild purgatives, such as cream of tartar, manna, senna or rhubarb.

When a bath cannot be had, six or eight bladders of hot water may do very well with the elder flower tea. If the putrid symptoms run high, bark may be depended on. One ounce in powder, with two drachms of Virginia snake-root, may be boiled in a pint of water, and a wine glass taken every hour, and apply a strong poultice of briony root or mustard to the feet; but unless a patient's blood before the attack be in a very bad state, and if the perspiration be attended to in the first instance, as it ought, there will be no fear of those dangerous symptoms. Should the elder flowers not be procurable, marsh-mallow roots, linseed, marygolds, balm, shepherd's purse, holy-thistle, sarsaparilla, viper-grass, and pimpernelle, will do as substitutes; but none are equal to the elder, fumitory and borage.

So convinced am I of the correctness of this mode of treatment, that nothing would give me greater pleasure than to see this system in practice; and much do I regret that it should not be introduced to the public by a much abler hand than mine. I leave the subject for the consideration of those who are showing the world every day that man is rising in intellect by thinking for himself. I should rejoice in having to defend this doctrine against combatants possessed of abilities and advantages sufficient to detect me if I had not truth and common sense on my side.

The monopoly of the profession has been for many years like a mill-stone about the neck of those who have a wish to make useful discovery in the cultivation, preparation, and employment of useful and natural remedies. There are more drugs swallowed in London alone than in the whole of Europe beside, four-fifths of which are either useless or pernicious; and my readers will perhaps be surprised to hear, that there are not less than thirty thousand medical men residing in London and its vicinity, who receive from the public, for coughs, colds, gout, consumption, fever, catarrhs, rheumatism, measles, small-pox, and accidents of "flood and field," (allowing each only £300 a year),about £9,464,000 per annum. This is a low calculation, for many could be named who are receiving from £3000 to £8000 a-year.

It is sufficient to point out these enormities to have the voices of the illiberal raised against me and my mode of practice; they find it their personal interest to support their order, and it is natural to expect from those who have devoted much of their time and attention to one particular course of treatment for all disorders and constitutions, that they should fall into the above error. They have a favourite child to nurse of their own, and they prefer it with the blind partiality of a parent. But am I singular in my opinions? By no means. The *Times* paper of 16th July 1831, says: *"We never read any reports where medical evidence is given without blushing for the state of medical science in England, and being convinced that this branch of education is defective, not only as regards the inculcation of sound principles, but even in the application of undoubted facts to recognized principles."* — And this confusion in the practice of medicine must remain so while the law confines it to certain licentiates, who all, with a very few exceptions, unite against any innovation, and who will make a greater stir in defending their exclusive privileges than they ever did or will in learning the healing art; the consequence has been, that the most eminent men, those who have conferred the greatest benefits on mankind, have had to encounter the greatest opposition from the faculty at large.

Harvey, who discovered the circulation of the blood, was branded as a quack and an impostor. John Hunter, who, like myself, spent the early part of his life as a tradesman, was attacked by the profession with all the ribaldry of vulgar insolence, although there is hardly a medical man in England but would feel it an honour to have known him. Dr. Jenner was treated and slandered in the same way, and had to seek refuge in the house of Colonel Watson, from the excited fury of the mob, set on by many of those very persons who would now consider it a great honour to be a Member of the Royal Jennerian Society. I could give the names of many other eminent men who have had to struggle with similar prejudices. Dr. Thornton is a living instance. Hear what he says of the liberality of his medical brethren. He states, that *"the small-pox is a disease too long known as productive of much emolument to all the branches of our profession; but every heart must pant to see this horrible disease banished from the earth; but, alas! instead of enquiry being steadily pursued and fair inductions made, an unexpected opposition arose, and the public were deluded by men who, to speak the least in their disfavour, should have known better; but on their account the people die. I have ventured to shew the torrent of their displeasure, and shall coolly investigate their several statements. I even trust and hope, finally, to see those same men at last adding to the glory of such noble example so honourable to the profession."*

Many of the profession speak against my treatment, as it takes good patients (as they are called) out of their hands, curing them and keeping them well. This resembles the objection the Assurance Offices had to Mr. Braithwaite's steam fire-engine - it extinguished the fires too expeditiously, as every great fire brought fresh customers to the office. The medical insurers of health act on the same principle. Sometimes their medicine shuts up the valves of vitality, and destroys the digestive powers of the stomach, which soon ends in death; and then to finish, if they hear that a man like myself has been in the room to visit as a friend or acquaintance, *"there is ground for a good cause against him."*

The following facts will serve as a specimen of the liberality of some men. About eighteen months since a gentleman, part of whose family had been under my care, called to consult me respecting a Gentleman residing in my parish. After hearing the particulars, I considered it beyond my ability; and not at any time wishing to interfere with the practice of medical men while there is any chance of their attendance doing good, and intending more over to confine myself to those complaints which I profess to understand, this feeling led me to decline attending; but after receiving several other applications, my friend told me I should oblige him by merely giving my opinion. I saw the helpless patient, only twenty-six years of age, completely bed-ridden, and given over by three of the most eminent Gentlemen in the metropolis, besides many others of inferior note, some of whom I knew to be very clever and good men. I felt myself imperatively called upon to act in this case, as I understood the nature of his complaint, and had a remedy for it; it was a glandular swelling, brought on by an affection of the spermatic cord. My treatment was fomentation, poultices, baths, and ointments externally; internal, teas or infusions of the most simple herbs, such as ground ivy, heart's-ease, briony, tormentil, cuckoo-point, &c. &c.

This gentleman walked to my house in Thayer Street within five weeks after this, and continues well. Now for the cream of the story. One of his physicians, on leaving him, begged of the patient, if he was ever fortunate enough to be cured, that the name of the practitioner should be sent to him, as he should most certainly introduce the case in one of his lectures. My patient, when perfectly cured, went to this gentleman's house. After the squeezing of hands and hearty congratulation on his wonderful recovery, this great man took his pen, and said: *"Now, Sir, for the name of the fortunate fellow who has done this wonder for you."* On my name being given, he said,

"Tilke! Tilke! why I never heard of his name in the profession before!". My patient replied, *"No, Sir; he is not a regular doctor, but was a tradesman in the neighbourhood where he now resides."* *"Oh!"* said this great man, *"I think I have heard of him before; I dare say it is that baker doctor who professes to cure the gout?"* The reply was, *"Yes, Sir, that is the man."* This had an instantaneous effect on this liberal man: he threw down the pen, and gave such restless tokens and signs to my poor patient as convinced him he had given great offence, in condescending to be cured by a quack.

I must confess I am not well acquainted with the meaning which the professional men have attached to the term of quackery; but I understand it to mean *mal-practice in physic*, or the exhibition of injurious or useless drugs for diseases of the human body, and that he who prescribes such injurious or useless a remedy is to all intents and purposes a quack. Then, I maintain, those gentlemen who attended this poor patient before me were all quacks, as they had all applied a useless remedy. I could not come under that name, as I applied *useful remedies* and cured the disease, which their best regular treatment now in practice had failed to do. Methinks I hear him telling one of his students, after my patient was let out, *"That fellow has suffered himself to be cured by a quack after I had given him up; it is enough to ruin my reputation. There is an unfeeling scoundrel for you! a man of honour would sooner have died under my hands. This must be put a stop to, or there's an end to all law and justice."*

Had I wished to avoid this contumely, what was to prevent me from purchasing a diploma, at the College of Aberdeen, Saint Andrew, Edinburgh, or Glasgow, where such things have been sold without the candidate being present? I say, had I cared for this mockery of common sense and understanding, I might have had my name and practice blazoned forth in the lecture-rooms, and in the medical publications of the day.-

> "For who shall go about
> To cozen fortune, and be honourable
> Without the stamp of merit! Let none presume
> To wear an undeserved dignity.
> Oh, that estates, degrees, and offices
> Were not derived corruptly! and that clear honour
> Were purchased by the merit of the wearer;
> How many then should cover that stand bare!
> How many be commanded that command!
> How much low peasantry would then be gleaned
> From the true seed of honour! And how much honour
> Picked from the chaff and ruin of the times
> To be new varnished."
>
> SHAKESPEAR.

How does this agree with the remarks of the liberal-minded Mr. Lawrence, who observes in one of his lectures, *"It is the obvious interest of the patient to be under the care of men who understand the case in all its bearings. It matters not,"* he says, *"to him whether he belongs to this or that college, or even if he belong to no college at all."* Doctor Burrows says, *"Medicine ever was and ever will be a conjectural science: the dogmas of schools are dangerous; because they are sanctioned by such an authority, and embraced unexamined, and perpetuated."* Dr. McCulloch observes, that it is quite time that physic should cease to *assert*, and commence to *prove*. "

TILKE'S CELEBRATED ESSENCES

OF

ALMOND, GINGER, ALLSPICE, CARRAWAY, CORIANDER,
CINNAMON, &c. &c.

are supplied to the Public, of the most superior qualities.
Sold in Two Ounce Bottles, at 2s, each.
The uses of these Essences, it is presumed, are too well
known to need description here. Suffice it to say,
that no Family who can afford it should be without
them.

Impurity of the Blood is the only Real
Disease to which Man is subject,

FOR WHICH TILKE'S

UNIVERSAL FAMILY PILLS

Are found so generally useful. The Inventor will prove, on oath, if required, that they do not contain one particle of mercurial or mineral substances, which are contrary to the natural constitution of man. They are composed of those tonic and bracing herbs, carduus benedictus, horehound, betony, coltsfoot, &c., and are strongly recommended for weak constitutions, especially after any severe fit of illness. They are also very beneficial for those females who lead a sedentary life, which relaxes the solids, enervates the mental powers, and disorders all the functions of the body. From the same cause proceed obstructions, indigestion, flatulence, and the whole train of nervous disorders, bringing on that painful state of the stomach which is described by the patient as peculiarly distressing, rivetting their attention, and poisoning all the sources of their enjoyment.

The success which has attended the use of these Pills, entitles them to the strongest recommendation, as they are found surprisingly efficacious in the above complaints, and they are found to be one of the best strengthening medicines and purifiers of the blood ever offered to the Public. Two, three, or four every night should be taken at the commencement, and the number gradually reduced.

TILKE'S GOUT PILLS,

To be taken while using the Ointment.

These pills are prepared from simple herbs; they do not contain one atom of either mercury, antimony, or the use of any drug what ever. Their first action is on the blood, therefore exercise promotes their good effects if taken as directed. With some constitutions they will not act on the bowels, in such cases they must take a little gentle opening medicine. These Pills stir up the humours, and evacuate such as the gout proceeds from; they greatly assist digestion, and cause the food to pass on to its respective parts for the purpose of supply to the system. The want of this effect is no doubt the first stage of gout, which may be known by a weakness and pain in the stomach, sickness, headache, giddiness, disrelish of food, sense of fullness after meals, spasms in the stomach, acidity, &c. These pills are to be taken one every four hours when the fit of the gout is on, and one every night at bed-time, to prevent the gout, assisted by soaking the feet and rubbing in the ointment once, and in very bad and long-standing cases twice a week. The proprietor pledges himself that these pills are mixed and made up with the most scrupulous accuracy, to accomplish which it has caused him many hours of intense study and practice, feeling and knowing how advantageous and essential it is in all diseases to adapt and combine medicines judiciously. No practitioner can do this unless he is the compounder of his medicine.

THE END.

LONDON:
Printed by J. Poulter, Great Chesterfield Street.

www.ingramcontent.com/pod-product-compliance
Lightning Source LLC
Chambersburg PA
CBHW082337290526
45793CB00008B/708